Psychological Self-Defense

To CANDACE,

KEEP BELIEVING,
REACH FOR THE STARS!

KEEP LEARNING,
KEEP GROWING!

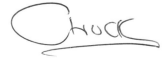

Copyright 2013 by Chuck O'Neill and Kate O'Neill

All Rights Reserved. No part of this book may be reproduced or utilized in any form or by any means, electronic or mechanical, including photocopying, without written permission from one of the authors.

Inquiries can be made at:

www.SifuChuck.com

Psychological Self-Defense

How to Protect Yourself from Predators, Criminals and Sociopaths <u>Before</u> They Attack

By

Sifu Chuck O'Neill

and

Kate O'Neill

Disclaimer

The principles in this book deal with self-defense—not attack or fighting. Fighting is illegal, and you can go to jail for breaking this law. Readers are responsible for knowing their own particular country, state, or provincial laws in regards to the use of excessive force, self-defense, and fighting. Neither the author nor the publisher assumes any responsibility for the use or misuse of the information contained in this book.

This book is not intended as legal advice and is not intended to replace getting professional, hands-on instruction in self-defense.

Table of Contents

Preface – A Note from the Authors 1

Chapter 1 – Why Psychological Self Defense?
(Or, How This Book Could Save Your Life!) 7

Chapter 2 – Anatomy of an Attack: Different Types of Attacks
and Attackers 18

Chapter 3 – Mastering the ABCs of Psychological Self Defense 29

Chapter 4 – Avoid Dangers before They Start: How to
Become an Awareness Super-Ninja 43

Chapter 5 – Listening to That Little Voice Inside:
The Survival Skill We All Naturally Have 61

Chapter 6 – The Predator Interview:
The Interview You DON'T Want to Pass 73

Chapter 7 – They Don't Think Like You: Understanding the
Mindset of a Predator 90

Chapter 8 – The Slow Poisoning of Sociopaths and
Narcissists in Your Life 107

Chapter 9 – Body Language: What Are You Saying to
People Around You? 126

Chapter 10 – What Are Other People Telling You?
Reading Others' Hidden Intentions through Their Body Language 140

Chapter 11 – How to Be a Human Lie Detector: Body Language
and Verbal Tells 156

Chapter 12 – How to Use Boundaries to Protect Yourself
from Predators 172

Chapter 13 – Confrontation: Using Visual and Verbal Skills to
Avoid an Attack 187

Chapter 14 – Physical Confrontations: What to Do
When All Else Fails 204

Chapter 15 – Finding Your Inner Warrior 215

About the Authors 220

Appendix A: Recommended Reading 222

Preface –
Psychological Self-Defense: A Note from the Authors

"Ultimate excellence lies not in winning every battle, but in defeating the enemy without ever fighting." — Sun Tzu, The Art of War

There are people out there who want to hurt you. They want to take what's yours. They want to control you. They want to see you suffer—sometimes emotionally, sometimes physically.

They may hurt you quickly, from out of the blue, or they may take their time and watch you, looking for a way to bring you down. But ultimately, they want to destroy you.

This book was written to help you stop them.

This book was written to help you protect yourself from those people—predators, criminals, sociopaths, liars, psychopaths, attackers, thieves, and narcissists.

As a martial arts instructor, self-defense teacher, bodyguard, and personal protection specialist, I've spent years teaching people how to protect themselves from predators.

And from my own experience—as well as the many stories people have shared with me—I've found that there are commonalities that precede most attacks.

The victims could have identified these commonalities if they had known about them. They could have been used to help the victims avoid attacks before they occurred.

And even if it had come down to a confrontation, there were still things the victims could have done—had they known about them—to avoid escalating the situation to a physical level.

That's the reason behind this book.

I want to give you the skills, tools, and knowledge you need to protect yourself from predators *before* they attack.

There are lots of experts teaching you what to do *when* you're attacked (self-defense courses, martial arts classes, etc.). This training is important.

However, nobody is talking about how to protect yourself *before* you're attacked.

Nobody is telling you how to identify predators, liars, and sociopaths who target you; how to send the messages that make them avoid choosing you as their next victim; or how to protect yourself so that you don't spend the rest of your life paying for what someone else did to you.

I wanted to put together the skills and tools you'll need to do this.

This group of tools, skills, and knowledge is what I have called *Psychological Self-Defense*. In my opinion, this is even more important to know than what to do when you are attacked because 95 percent of the time, I believe that it's possible to avoid the actual attack in the first place. And it's a heck of a lot easier than dealing with an attack after it's happened.

Dealing with an attack—even if you come out the 'winner'—is devastating and difficult. There will be physical, emotional, and mental wounds that will need to heal. There might even be legal repercussions. It could affect your life for years to come in ways you could never have imagined.

So, if you could learn some skills, some tools to place in your *Psychological Self-Defense* arsenal, wouldn't it be worth it do so?

I want to help you avoid becoming a victim in the first place, using what you'll learn in this book.

Please note, however, I didn't write this book to make you fear the outside world; 99 percent of the people you come across mean you no harm.

This book is about the 1 percent that could be a problem.

I hope that by reading this book you will feel more confident and prepared to handle whatever—and whomever—life throws at you.

Sifu Chuck O'Neill, www.SifuChuck.com

Being married to a man who lives, breathes, and sleeps personal security has been an eye-opening experience for me. I discovered early on in our marriage that my husband could go from a dead sleep, flat on his back, to fully upright and alert on the bed, ready to attack in two seconds flat. (It makes you think twice about cuddling!)

While it's fascinating to be with a man who can spot a shoplifter, mugger, or thief from a mile away, the most compelling part of it all for me has been the stories—stories from Chuck's students, coworkers, and the people at his self-protection seminars.

Many of these stories have been heartbreaking. But many of them have also been inspiring—stories of people who have used many of the principles you will learn in this book, people who refused to become victims and fought back to triumph over their attackers.

As someone who has made a lifelong study of human psychology, body language, and behavior, the human spirit never ceases to amaze me with its resilience and tenacity. We truly don't know how strong we really are.

There was one common theme to these stories, however, that I noticed over the years. Without exception, after an attack people always asked Chuck the same question: "What could I have done to prevent this?"

Nine times out of ten, there was always something they could have done to avoid the confrontation—had they known, had they been given the right tools.

That is why I'm so proud that Chuck has chosen to share the tools in this book and that he's asked me to contribute my knowledge of human psychology and body language to help round out the information.

Most chapters will be written from Chuck's perspective. However, a few that deal with the psychology of the predator, body language, and lying are a joint effort from both of us. In those instances, you will see which author's perspective (Chuck's or mine) you're reading in order to make it easier to understand.

Also, please note that while the stories you'll read in this book are true, some of the names and unimportant details have been changed to protect the dignity and reputation of the people involved.

Thank you for taking the time to read Psychological Self-Defense. It's my hope that you will find this book educational, entertaining, and lifesaving.

Kate O'Neill, H.BSc. www.BodyLanguageMatters.com

Chapter 1 –
Why *Psychological Self-Defense?* (Or, How This Book Could Save Your Life!)

By Chuck O'Neill

> "... there are at least 2 million psychopaths in North America ... Consider also that the prevalence of psychopathy in our society is about the same as that of schizophrenia ..."
> — Robert D. Hare, Without Conscience
> —The Disturbing World of Psychopaths Among Us

> "Statistics show that a woman now 21 years old has a 1 in 4 chance of experiencing a violent crime in her lifetime." — AWARE.org

> "1 in 25 ordinary Americans secretly has no conscience and can do anything at all without feeling guilty." — Martha Stout, The Sociopath Next Door

A Not-So-Great Example of Psychological Self-Defense:

It was 1999, Montego Bay, Jamaica. And we were in serious trouble.

The man with the dreadlocks and the six-inch straight razor was now moving in behind my wife. He eyed Kate intensely, hungrily taking in her pale white skin and long red hair.

Completely oblivious to the unfolding situation, Kate stumbled along behind me as we walked single file down the narrow, crowded sidewalk. She clung to my hand, letting me lead her into what I now realized was an elegantly set trap.

The man's partner, who'd approached me about thirty seconds earlier, walked backwards in front of me. He was attempting to distract me with his fast talk and friendly jokes.

There was very little time to act. I turned and scanned the street beside us. A car was coming up the street and blocking our escape—but we would have a window in about twenty seconds.

I switched my grip and clamped down on Kate's hand, strengthening the hold I had on her. The man with the dreadlocks was now about three feet away, pushing people aside and closing in fast. The man in front of me grew louder and more animated as he saw his partner moving into place. We were effectively being herded into position.

It was now or never.

As the car passed, giving me an opening, I whipped around ninety degrees and bolted out into the street, dragging my poor, shocked wife along behind me.

People stared as we sprinted up the street and in the opposite direction of the two men targeting us, weaving in and out of moving cars like a couple of insane asylum escapees.

I could hear my wife behind me as I pulled her along. "What the heck are you doing? Where are we going? I thought we wanted to go that way!"

She was pointing back the way we came. I barked back at her, "Don't ask questions! Just keep going!"

I could feel the adrenaline coursing through me as we reached the top of the hill, back to the tourist bus that had brought us to the market area.

I looked back, but the two men hadn't followed us. The man with the dreadlocks was still where we'd left him, his eyes now on me, assessing the situation. He then turned to his partner and raised his hands as if to say, "What happened?" His partner was red faced and clearly swearing up a storm, incensed at having lost their prey so easily.

A moment later, Dreadlocks ambled back across the street to his original post where I'd first noticed him watching us, probably getting the trap ready for the next naive tourist to come his way.

As we made our way back towards the bus, I overheard a female police officer arguing with one of our fellow tourists.

"No, sir—you CAN'T go down that way. That street is not safe for tourists. You need to stay up here, sir. Stay in this area."

I almost laughed. Where had she been ten minutes ago when I'd wandered down that way and almost led my wife into a trap?

I now had to figure out a way to explain to Kate why I'd nearly ripped her arm off a second ago. She stood glaring at me, rubbing her arm and waiting for an explanation from her crazy husband.

"Come on, honey, I'll buy you a coffee before we hit the bus." I smiled sheepishly. Maybe a little caffeine would put her in a better mood, considering I now had to explain what had almost just happened to her.

Just so you know—this is NOT a good example of psychological self-defense. I made a lot of mistakes in that situation that could have been deadly, mistakes you'll learn not to make in this book.

But it's also a great example of how—even if you do make a mistake and end up in a red-flag situation—you can use your psychological self-defense to turn it around and protect yourself.

So What Exactly IS Psychological Self-Defense Anyway?

Psychological self-defense is a set of skills you can use to protect yourself ahead of time and avoid becoming a victim in the first place. Many people will tell you what to do to defend yourself when you're attacked, but why not avoid the attack in the first place?

Psychological self-defense is the easiest way to protect yourself from predators, criminals, and sociopaths *before* they attack. It's far easier to head off a possible attack before it happens when you use some simple principles of human behavior and psychology.

Every experienced martial artist and security professional will tell you that the best thing you can do to defend yourself in a fight is to avoid it in the first place.

Think of psychological self-defense as smart preventative measures you can use to avoid that confrontation—to avoid becoming a victim in the first place.

> *"Self Defense is primarily not being there when the other guy wants to fight."*
> — Lawrence A. Kane and Kris Wilder,
> The Little Black Book of Violence

Don't get me wrong, there's tremendous value in learning martial arts or taking a self-defense class. As a martial arts instructor and personal protection specialist, I teach people every day how to physically defend themselves and disable an attacker.

However, a lot of people just don't have the time or the inclination to spend hours learning a martial art. And, because of the mind-numbing effects of adrenaline, they may find it hard—if not impossible—to remember their intricate self-defense moves when faced with an attack.

But what they can do is learn the principles of psychological self-defense that we lay out in this book to protect themselves from danger ahead of time.

What Will You Learn from This Book?

In this book you're going to learn simple, easy, doable principles that will help prevent about 95 percent of the harmful situations you may face in your lifetime.

You're going to learn how to be empowered when you face unsafe people or situations. (And you'll also learn what to do in those rare situations when you face danger that you could *not* have prevented.)

You're going to learn:

◊ How to be **A**ware of potential problems before they start—and see them coming when nobody else does.

◊ How to use your **B**ody language and **B**oundaries to protect yourself.

◊ And how to use verbal and visual **C**onfrontation skills to de-escalate a tense situation.

I call these the ABCs of psychological self–defense: Awareness, Boundaries and Body Language, and Confrontation (verbal, visual, and finally physical).

You'll learn simple skills that you can put into practice, skills you can use to avoid not only physical attacks, but also more subtle, emotional and covert psychological attacks as well.

After we're done, you'll have the tools to feel more confident, powerful, and in control of your personal safety.

An Ounce of Prevention...

Practicing psychological self-defense is very similar to practicing cancer prevention. It's so much easier to prevent cancer by taking simple steps every day than it is to get cancer and then have to face treatment. (Eating your cancer-fighting blueberries every day is a whole lot easier and more enjoyable than going through chemo and radiation once you have cancer.)

In a similar way, the principles in this book are much easier to practice than getting to the stage where you become the victim of a predator, have to defend yourself from an attacker, or pick up the pieces of your life after it's been shattered by a sociopath.

So why not do the easy thing now to protect yourself? Why not take small measures every day and avoid facing the harsh end-stage results of an attack on yourself or your family?

Because I teach martial arts, I hear a lot of unfortunate stories from people who have been through an attack before they come to train with me. I also hear stories of my current students using their martial arts skills to defend themselves in physical confrontations.

And I have to tell you, these are not happy stories.

Even if someone 'wins' a fight or they're successful in defending themselves using their martial arts skills, they often still have to deal with injuries and trauma after the fact.

And do you know the number one question they ask me?

"Sifu, what could I have done differently?"

They all want to know how they could have prevented the attack in the first place. They aren't happy they were attacked (even though they may have won the fight).

Every single one of them—without exception—would have chosen to *avoid* the attack in the first place.

Here's the thing though: In every single case I've come across, most of them—about 95 percent—could have been avoided by using the principles of *Psychological Self-Defense*. Unfortunately, most people did not know these principles at the time. That's the main reason I wrote this book.

I speak regularly to groups on personal protection and self-defense. And it amazes me how many people don't have a clue how to protect themselves with these principles. But they need to know—more now than ever—how to defend themselves and how to protect their lives and their families from predators.

Where Can You Use Psychological Self-Defense?

You can use the principles you'll learn in this book to defend and protect yourself against physical attackers—muggers, rapists, criminals, home invaders, and more.

But you can also use them for so much more.

You can use them to help you in everyday situations to protect yourself from people who want to do you harm—not just physically, but emotionally and mentally as well:

- ◊ the jealous coworker who wants to destroy your reputation and steal your job
- ◊ the next-door neighbour who leers at you every time you're out gardening
- ◊ the handsome 'charmer' who's really just trolling for a sugar-mama to sponge off for the rest of his life
- ◊ the business partner who plans to swindle you out of a multi-million-dollar deal
- ◊ the 'charismatic leader' who's nothing but a sociopath in disguise looking for another victim to join his cult
- ◊ the con artist who plans to steal your identity and drain your bank accounts

◊ the attractive woman who targets you for an affair but is really a honey-trap stealing your company's secrets

◊ the narcissistic 'friend' who takes and takes, draining you dry and confusing you with their passive-aggressive mind games

Basically, there are so many ways you can use the principles in this book, not just to protect yourself, but to actually improve your life and attain more of what you want.

Using these principles, you'll also learn to identify 'safe people' (who will enrich your life in numerous ways) versus 'unsafe people'.

You'll be able to read people's unspoken intentions and pick up on undercurrents you never realized were there before. You'll be able to de-escalate tense situations and persuade people to do things your way.

You'll have the edge in everything from your dating life to your business life.

What This Book Is NOT

I realize that in the world of self-defense and personal protection, there is a lot of fear. Please know: This is not a fear-mongering book. It's not intended to turn you into a suspicious, neurotic basket-case peering anxiously around every corner for the next potential predator.

I'm not a fear-monger. I don't believe in scaring people to get a reaction, to get noticed, or to sell books.

But I am a realist. I won't sugarcoat things to give you the warm fuzzies, telling you that you'll never face a predator or an attack situation.

Because that's not reality either.

Reality is seeing the world as it really is—not hiding from it, but not making it worse than it is either.

And the reality is that there are bad people out there. The reality is that with all the people you meet in your life, you have a 100 percent chance of running into at least one of them, if not several.

That's the reality. But it's also reality to say that these predators are a very small portion of the population. At any one time, about 1 to 5 percent of the population is made up of predators, emotionally disturbed people, or sociopaths.

So the truth is that they are out there—but they're in the minority.

And if you use the skills in this book, you are much less likely to come across them or trigger them to attack you personally.

Most people are good, kind, and generally act in accordance with the accepted laws of polite society. They may lie occasionally, or gossip, or act selfishly. We all do. But these are not dangerous people. And they aren't out to get you.

This book is not about those people. It's about the rare group who *are* out to harm you. It's about knowing what to do when you come across them. It's about knowing that you have the power to protect yourself should you become a target.

Fairy-Tale Fear vs. Logical Fear

There are two different types of fear: fairy-tale fear and logical fear. You have to know the difference.

Fairy-tale fear is fabricated and comes usually from reading too many fear-mongering books or watching the sensationalist news media (which can make you believe that everyone is out to mug you, lie to you, or steal from you).

Fairy-tale fear isn't real. But it can harm you.

It can make you look for boogeymen in every closet or down every dark alley. It can make you paranoid. It can cause you to lose out on your life and avoid taking the necessary risks that will get you ahead. And it will torment you.

That's not the kind of fear I want you to have; it's not based in reality.

What you want to have is logical fear—a healthy knowledge of reality—knowing that danger exists and that you may, one day, run into it. It's having a healthy respect for a potentially dangerous situation while knowing you can take steps to protect yourself before this situation turns ugly.

It's not sticking your head in the sand, but it's also not turning a paper cut into multiple stab wounds.

Logical fear will keep you sane—and safe. Logical fear keeps you empowered and in control at all times. And that's what will keep you alive.

Important Points:

- ◊ *Psychological Self-Defense* is a set of skills you can use to stop attacks before they happen.

- ◊ While it's important to know how to defend yourself should you get into a physical altercation, it's more important to know how to avoid the attack in the first place.

- ◊ The ABCs of *Psychological Self-Defense* are: Awareness, Body Language and Boundaries, and Confrontation—verbal, visual, and physical.

- ◊ *Psychological Self-Defense* is like cancer prevention; it's easier and more enjoyable to practice than dealing with the end results of not practicing it.

- ◊ You can use *Psychological Self-Defense* in multiple ways, not just to protect yourself from physical attacks. You can use it to protect yourself from emotional and psychological predators and to improve your life overall.

◊ You must learn to discern between fairy-tale fear and logical fear.

◊ Fairy-tale fear is not based in reality and will take over your life and torment you.

◊ Logical fear is having a realistic view of the world, respecting potentially dangerous situations, and knowing you are prepared to handle them.

Chapter 2 –
Anatomy of an Attack: Different Types of Attacks and Attackers

By Chuck O'Neill

"Know Your Enemy" – Sun Tzu

"Hell, I'll kill a man in a fair fight ... or if I think he's gonna start a fair fight ... or if he bothers me ... or if there's a woman ... or if I'm gettin' paid ... mostly only when I'm gettin' paid."
–Mal, Firefly (TV Series)

When people talk about being attacked, they're usually referring to being attacked physically, like when someone jumps you, beats you, and steals your wallet. Or when you're in a bar and a guy picks a fight with you and cracks you in the jaw.

But there are actually different types of attacks. In fact, you might be getting attacked right now and not even know it!

In order to understand how to properly apply the skills you'll learn in this book, you have to understand the different types of attacks. That way, you'll understand which skills to apply and when to apply them. Because the skills that may work in one type of attack may not work in a different type of attack.

The Four Different Types of Attacks:

#1: Physical: This is when someone attacks you physically, as in the examples above. Their aim is to physically harm or disable you in order to take something from you.

Criminals, thieves, rapists, and home invaders fall into this category. These kinds of attacks can involve a high level of physical violence.

#2: Emotional/Psychological: This is when someone attacks you emotionally and psychologically. They play with your head, destroy your confidence, suck you dry financially, manipulate you into giving them more than you want to, and leave you an emotional wreck.

This may involve verbal abuse as well. Psychopaths, cult leaders, identity thieves, narcissists, and con artists fall into this category. These kinds of attacks may seem less harmful on the surface; however, their damage can run even deeper than physical attacks.

#3: Overt Attacks: This is when someone is clearly gunning for you. That nasty coworker accuses you of stealing from the company in front of the entire office. That moron in the bar is coming straight for you.

These are clear, outright attacks, and they often do end up in the confrontation stage if they are not prevented ahead of time.

#4: Covert Attacks: These are when you don't know someone is gunning for you—until the damage has been done.

For example, you apply for a home mortgage and discover that your identity was stolen two years ago by that 'great guy' you met at the gym; you wake up one day and realize that the business venture you invested in was a fraud perpetrated by a local con artist, and now you're broke.

Covert attacks may not end up in the confrontation stage; it's usually too late for that by the time you realize what's happened to you. However, with the skills you'll learn in this book, you can spot the signs ahead of time and take steps to avoid being attacked in this way.

Most attacks are a mix of #1 or #2 and #3 or #4. For example, my Jamaican experience from chapter one was a ***physical, covert attack*** (or it would have been if I had fallen into the trap).

A guy who takes a swing at you in a bar for eyeing his girlfriend is an example of a ***physical, overt attack.*** (You can easily see it coming from a mile away; he's not trying to hide it.)

A narcissistic boss who insults you in front of the entire office to make himself look better is an example of an ***emotional, overt attack.***

A jealous friend who tells the guy of your dreams that you have herpes is an example of an ***emotional, covert attack.*** (You probably won't even know it happened; you'll just wonder why the guy stopped calling you.)

Another thing to realize is that attacks can easily change. For example, a verbal, emotional attack can quickly escalate to a physical attack. A covert attack can turn into an overt attack if you start to realize what the other person is trying to do to you.

The important thing here is to realize that there are different ways in which people can attack you.

And just as with physical self-defense, where there is no one move that will work every time, there is no one right move in Psychological Self-Defense that will work in every type of attack. You have to consider the type of attack you're dealing with first.

You also have to consider the type of attacker.

Five Different Types of Attackers

In different attack situations, there are also different types of attackers. Sometimes you have the luxury of knowing what type of attacker you're dealing with. Other times you don't.

But just so you're aware, we're going to go over the most common types of attackers here. This is because, as with different types of attacks, different attackers may require a different response from you.

#1: The In-Your-Face Attacker: This is your basic criminal who jumps you from the bushes and demands your wallet or tries to beat you up. You could also call this guy the 'anonymous' attacker, because you know absolutely nothing about him.

Chances are you've never seen him before and didn't see him coming. This kind of attacker usually initiates a physical, covert and/or overt attack.

#2: The Sociopathic Attacker: The sociopath has no conscience and will literally destroy your life for the fun of watching it go 'boom'. They can be criminals (and therefore, physically violent).

However, many of them are too smart to do anything worth jail time (and get caught). They may appear to be magnetic and popular. Many cult leaders are sociopaths.

A sociopath—whether physically violent or not—is not easily talked down. Their goal is worth everything to them and they'll do anything to reach it.

They can't be reasoned with. And because they feel no guilt, they really don't care if you catch them in a lie or a covert attack.

There will be no remorse from these people, and often the only way to protect yourself is to get away from them. We'll be dedicating several chapters to exploring this type of predator along with attacker type #3.

#3: The Narcissist or Other Personality Disordered Attacker: This person—unlike the sociopath—does have a conscience. However, they often choose to ignore it and hurt you anyway. But they will try to cover it up because they do realize that what they've done is wrong, and if you confront them, they may back down in order to save face.

These types of predators tend to be more subtle and initiate more covert, psychological attacks on their victims.

However, like the sociopath, they can be very destructive and not easily reasoned with. They may get off on all the drama you create if you confront them, so they actually like it if you create more.

#4: The Everyday, Dumbass Attacker: This guy is not a criminal. He's not a sociopath or even a narcissist. He's just a dumbass.

He might be that guy in the bar who wants to show off to his friends by planting your face in the table. He might be the drunk at a football game who doesn't agree with your choice of team—and shows you the error of your ways with his fist.

It might be the Paris Hilton wannabe who doesn't like the way her boyfriend is smiling at you. So she decides to rip out your hair extensions instead of kicking his ass.

This kind of attacker is probably not thinking and is fairly easy to see coming. They aren't as evil or cunning as the predators above.

They might just be the wrong person in the wrong circumstances. These people can often be talked down because, at the heart of it, they really don't want trouble either.

#5: The Physically Driven Attacker: This guy is strongly physically driven in some way. Mainly, we're talking here about people under the influence of drugs—legal and illegal.

For example, this kind of attacker might be going through heroin withdrawal and is thus willing to do whatever it takes to get a fix. Or she may be desperate for codeine and willing to break into your home and dig through your medicine cabinet to get it.

The one word to describe the physically driven attacker is 'desperate'. They will often do anything—anything—to get what they need.

They may be completely nice, wonderful people were it not for the substance that they so desperately need. Under the influence, however, they become completely different people. That's how, for example, a sweet little girl who used to call you 'Mommy' can now take a knife and come at your throat as a drugged-out teen.

Because these attackers are physically driven, chances are you won't be able to talk them down. They aren't even able to think logically.

Your best bet is to see them coming and avoid them altogether. If you do get into a confrontation with these attackers, you need to realize they will do insane things that don't make any sense in order to get their fix.

A physical take-down may be the only way to stop them if you can't avoid them. You may also have to put up boundaries to stop them.

So those are five different types of attackers. It's important to know what you're dealing with—if possible—in every attack situation. Because then you'll know which psychological self-defense tools are the best ones to use.

What Happens to You When You're Physically Attacked?

Do you actually know what happens to you when you're in an attack or confrontation situation? Most people don't. But it's important to know so that you aren't taken by surprise.

Kate experienced firsthand what happens when people face attack situations one morning a few months ago.

I'd said good-bye on my way out the door, but, unbeknownst to her, I stopped to answer some e-mails in my office. Then I went downstairs to the basement to pack up some gear for a class I was teaching that morning.

Kate was in the kitchen and had heard the alarm signal. So she assumed she was alone in the house and that I'd set the alarm on my way out.

We'd had several break-and-enters in our neighbourhood that month, so she was already a bit on edge. Then she heard the noises downstairs.

She ignored what she heard at first as the house we were in could be creaky at times. But then she heard them again.

Her blood ran cold and her heart started to race as she heard heavy steps coming up the basement stairs.

(Our house at the time did have one vulnerability—the basement. There was a glass door in the basement that someone could easily break and step through to enter the home without sounding the alarm. She told me later that this was exactly what she thought had happened.)

Kate peered around the kitchen door through our dining room to the stairs, but all she saw was a man in black (me in my black jacket and toque). She literally froze until a few minutes later when I walked into view and she saw my face.

Within seconds Kate was shaking and breaking down in tears as the stress of the situation melted away. The funny thing was that when she really thought she was facing a home invasion, she'd frozen. She admitted later that her mind had gone completely blank.

She couldn't think. She had picked up a knife from the counter but had completely forgotten about it until I cautiously pointed out that she was still holding it.

She also realized after the fact that she'd been standing right beside the kitchen door that led out to the backyard. Her escape was just three steps away, but she hadn't even thought to run out the door. Her mind had shut down, and the ability to see an easy escape route had not occurred to her.

Kate's not unique in this regard. In an attack situation almost everyone freezes and their brain shuts down.

"The stress of a crisis can cause the key part of the brain that processes new information to misfire. People lose their ability to make decisions. They turn into statues." — Ben Sherwood, The Survivors Club, The Secrets and Science that Could Save Your Life

This is why I don't recommend fancy, intricate self-defense classes for people, especially if they aren't willing to continually train the techniques. Because in an adrenaline-fueled situation, you won't be able to remember them.

When I teach self-defense moves, I try to make them so simple that people can remember at least one of them in a crisis situation. That's also why people who take martial arts are continually training their techniques over and over again. So that when they have to use them to defend themselves, they know them cold.

The plain truth is, however, that most people these days just don't have the time to train in self-defense or martial arts every week.

That's why the best defense is spotting an attack ahead of time so that you can avoid it.

We'll be learning just how to do that in the next chapter with the ABCs of psychological self-defense.

Freeze, Fight, or Flight

The 'Fight or Flight' process was first coined by Walter Cannon, a Harvard psychologist. It was later expanded to include the 'Freeze' response also. Knowing about this survival response you naturally have inside of you will help you to understand what happens when you find yourself in a highly stressful situation.

This survival response has been developed over thousands of years. Long before grocery stores, we had to hunt for our food. And in many cases early man could move from predator to prey in seconds. As part of that response to high levels of stress, we developed the 'Freeze, Flight, or Fight' instincts that dump chemicals like adrenaline into our bloodstream when facing danger.

Regardless of who we are, our first natural reaction to the sign of danger is the 'freeze' response. This may be for only a second, but it still happens to all of us. Everyone freezes.

This is partially because we hope we aren't seen or noticed by the predator. It's also our brain's way of assessing the situation. We may also stay in this mode if we feel that fleeing or fighting are not viable alternatives.

Over the years of training and teaching, I have found that having a 'command word' has always helped me move from freeze to either fight or flight. I've found it works exceptionally well when under high stress or even when I've been dazed in sparring. You may want to choose and practice using your own command word.

For example, my command word is 'Go'. Simple, direct, commanding. I may not need to scream it out loud, but I know when my brain is ordering me to 'go'.

Our next natural response is actually to 'flee'. Our self-survival instinct kicks in, and all we want to do is run and 'live to fight another day'. When you do flee, don't be ashamed of it. Your body has determined that the risks are too great to stay around.

The last response is 'fight'. In many cases this occurs when we don't feel we have any options, such as being cornered, or we feel that we can definitely dominate our opponent. In today's society, the aggressive 'fight' response can even show up in boardroom negotiations and arguments with significant others.

One of the best examples of the fight response came in a story I heard of a woman whose car was stolen while she was getting gas. Her six-month-old child was in the back seat when the carjacker started to drive away.

This woman literally jumped into the driver's side window and fought with the carjacker while he was trying to drive away. The carjacker lost control of the car and ran away. Talk about the true 'Momma Bear' fighting instinct kicking in!

Know that the Freeze, Flight, or Fight response is normal. The more aware you are of this response, the more you will start to recognize it occurring in your everyday life when you're highly stressed. With time and practice you will be able to work with your natural survival system instead of against it.

Important Points:

◊ Not every attack is the same. In order to know how to protect yourself, you have to know what kind of attack and attacker you're facing.

◊ There are four different types of attacks: physical, emotional/psychological, covert, and overt. These can be a mix and can even shift from one type of attack into another.

◊ There are five main kinds of attackers: the sudden, in-your-face attacker; the sociopathic attacker; the narcissistic attacker; the dumbass, everyday attacker; and the physically driven attacker.

◊ Knowing what kind of attacker you're facing (if possible) will help you decide how to defend and protect yourself.

◊ Most people, when faced with a confrontation or attack situation, will freeze for a time. They will not be able to think clearly or remember complicated self-defense moves.

◊ Your best form of protection is to use the ABCs of psychological self-defense to stop an attack before it happens.

Chapter 3 –
Mastering the ABCs of Psychological Self-Defense

By Chuck O'Neill

Kevin's Story:

Kevin is a student at a downtown university. He's just finished his last exam for the first term. He's exhausted, but he's happy that it's finally over.

His friends have razzed him mercilessly about having his final test on the last day of exams—just his luck. Almost everyone on campus has cleared out for the holiday season while Kevin had to wait. But that was all over now.

He turns his exam in and goes out into the hallway, sighing with relief.

He packs up his bag, puts on his coat, and walks out into the freezing winter night air. Just one last stop at his dorm to pick up his things and he's out of there. He can hardly wait.

The campus looks strangely deserted with everyone gone, like a snow-covered ghost town lost in shadows.

A bit unnerved, Kevin takes his iPod out of his pocket and sticks his earphones into his ears. He decides to play the new songs he downloaded from iTunes that day. The sounds of his feet crunching through the snow as he trudges across the campus are soon drowned out by Usher's latest song.

An ice-cold wind sends shivers down his back. *Man, it's freezing*. He should have brought his hat and gloves. He should have worn his long underwear. He should have worn a parka—or two.

Trying to keep his mind off the cold, Kevin looks down at his feet and hunches his shoulders to preserve body heat. Doesn't help.

Suddenly a stab of pain explodes through his skull and stars dance in front of his eyes as he staggers and falls, leaving a pool of blood staining the pristine white snow.

Salma's Story:

Salma is on vacation at a five-star resort in Mexico with her best friend, Stacey. They're having the time of their lives, sunning themselves by the pool, sipping margaritas, and dancing until dawn every night.

They're both hot, blond, and single—and they know how to get a man's attention. There's no shortage of men vying for them back home in New York, and the men in Cancun are no different.

Every night they enjoy free drinks, admiring looks, and compliments galore. This is the best vacation of Salma's life. She feels on top of the world. She can't wait for the party in the hotel cantina tonight—it's going to be hot.

That night Salma's friend Stacey meets Juan, a young Antonio Banderas look-alike. They dirty dance and flirt heavily all night. The man is clearly high-class all the way: He's sporting a large gold Rolex, a tailored suit, and, according to Stacey, he drives a new fire-engine red Lamborghini.

The best news, Stacey tells Salma, is that Juan is actually a local who's doing some business at the resort. He's offered to show the two girls around town the next day and take them to where the real action is, where the locals go for a good time.

Salma feels a twinge of doubt. "But we don't really know him, Stace. I don't know…"

"Come oooooooonnnnn," Stacey groans, flopping on the bed in her usual, overly dramatic way. "He's hot, rich, and driving a sweet car. What more do you need to know?"

She pouts at Salma. "Don't be a stick-in-the-mud. We're on vacation. Let's live a little. Don't you want to see where the locals go? After all, Juan will be with us the whole time. We'll be safe."

Salma looks at her friend, now on her knees on the bed in a mock-begging pose. She smiles. "Okay—but only for a few hours this afternoon. Tell him we have to be back at the hotel for dinner."

Stacey hops up, squeals, and goes to call Juan. She returns later, floating on a cloud of blissful infatuation. Juan will pick them up in an hour in front of the hotel lobby.

Salma and Stacey disappear that night and are never heard from again.

Chris's Story:

Chris and his girlfriend Tina both had a rough week at work. To blow off some steam, they decide to head out to their local pub on a Friday night.

A couple of friends cancel out on them at the last minute, so it's just the two of them. They decide to relax over a few drinks and then head home.

Halfway through their drinks, Chris strikes up a conversation with two guys at the table next to them. They seem friendly enough, so he invites them to come and drink at their table.

They both pull up chairs and order another round of drinks.

The two guys, Carl and Mike, work in construction. They entertain Chris and Tina for nearly two hours with stories of all the crazy stunts they pull at their job sites. Chris orders another round on him, and his two new best friends slap him on the back to say thanks.

Tina excuses herself to go to the bathroom and the conversation lulls. Chris notices Carl and Mike watching Tina leave. They clearly appreciate a good-looking woman.

"Your girl is really cute." Carl grins.

Chris smiles. Guys will be guys. "Yeah, she is."

He's not upset. After all, they can look, but he's the one going home with her.

The guys start talking about the latest MMA fight. Chris is feeling pretty buzzed and joins in where he can although he doesn't really know a lot about the subject.

These guys are clearly fanatics though. They even get up and start pantomiming the high points of the latest fight with each other. Chris laughs. It's fun to watch two huge, drunk idiots stumbling around acting like they're famous MMA fighters.

Tina returns to the table and joins in the party, hooting, clapping, and cheering them on. The guys pick up their game for her, like peacocks strutting for the prize.

Finally exhausted, they crash down in their seats, happy to knock back the latest round.

Mike turns to Tina.

"You know, you're pretty hot. You a model?"

Tina laughs. "Not now—but I used to be."

Mike winks at her. "You ever do nude photos? I got a buddy who takes nudes of girls like you. Bet I could get him to take a few—you might even make some cash at it."

Shifting in her chair, Tina gives him a tight smile. "No, I'm not interested—but thanks anyway."

Ignoring her, Carl chimes in, "I bet you'd look great naked."

Mike laughs. "Now there's a visual I could go for."

Chris feels slightly uncomfortable but laughs along anyway. He suddenly doesn't like the way Mike and Carl are eyeing his girlfriend.

"Hey, man," Chris says, trying to turn the heat down a bit. "She said she's not interested. Let it go."

"Whatever, dude, just saying why not—she's half-dressed now anyway. What's a little more skin? Come on, honey. Ever done a table dance?" Mike thumps on the table, gesturing to Tina to get up and give it a go.

Tina is clearly uncomfortable. "Chris..."

"Hey, guys, enough." Chris orders angrily. "That's not okay."

Mike and Carl look at each other. Chris can see the gears in their heads turning. Two guys against one...

It was time to leave. "I think we need to get going anyway."

"Yeah," Tina catches on and chimes in, "I have to get up early for work tomorrow, so maybe it's time to go."

She looks around the bar nervously. Chris follows her eyes. The bar is practically empty—the four of them have stayed until closing time. Chris tries to get up casually and put his jacket on.

"Thanks guys, it was fun. I'll get that last round. Maybe we'll see you again sometime."

"What's the hurry? You can't leave now," Carl smiles but it doesn't quite reach his eyes. He looks at Tina. "We were just gettin' to know each other."

This time, there's no mistaking his intention.

Chris picks up Tina's jacket and helps her put it on, his mind now racing, trying to figure out how he can get out of this one. He's been in bar fights before. He knows where this is going.

"Thanks, but my girl here is tired and we have an early day tomorrow. You guys have a good night."

Carl slams his fist on the table, red-faced, his temperature rising.

"I SAID you can't leave now. You think you're the man? Just cuz we had a bit of fun with your girl here? What kind of drinking buddy are you anyway?"

Mike chimes in, "I think you're right Carl, this guy thinks he's better than us." He looks at Chris. "You're turning into a giant asshole, man. I say you need a lesson in manners."

Chris gently pushes Tina away from the table and turns to face the two guys. They're drunk and riled—and not likely to be talked down now that their egos are on the line.

They both rise to face Chris. Mike makes a fist with his right hand and then lets it go, only to make it again.

Chris glances at Tina, who nervously chews her lip and scans furtively for anyone who could step in and help them. "Tina, go get the bartender."

As Chris watches her leave, he's too late to see the first punch being thrown his way. The last sounds he hears are Tina's screams as he stumbles back before hitting the floor.

Psychological Self-Defense—the ABCs

All three of these stories show you examples of where psychological self-defense could have been used to avoid an attack. However, they're all very different stories.

For example, Kevin's attack was covert and physical. Salma and Stacey's attack was covert and psychological (at least at the start when Juan was persuading them to go with him). Chris's attack was overt and physical.

Their attackers were also very different.

Kevin's attacker was an in-your-face, anonymous attacker. Salma and Stacey's attacker was a sociopath working for a sex-trafficking ring. Chris's predators were just dumbass, everyday attackers.

So how do you come up with a defense system that covers all of these situations?

In teaching personal protection, I wanted to come up with an easy way for people to understand the order of how attacks proceed. I also wanted to teach a basic strategy that people could easily remember in any type of dangerous situation.

The result was the ABCs of psychological self-defense.

These are, as you've already read: Awareness, Body Language and Boundaries, and Confrontation—verbal and visual tactics. This is a simple way to remember how to defend yourself in any dangerous situation.

They are also in this order to help you understand that attacks are progressive.

Attacks Are Progressive

For example, the easiest way to avoid an attack is at the 'A'— or Awareness—stage. The second stage is the Body language and Boundaries stage. The last stage is Confrontation, and trouble is a lot harder to avoid once you've reached that stage (but not impossible).

So if you can shut things down at the Awareness or initial Body language stage, your odds of getting out of an attack are much better than if you reach the later Confrontation stage.

Reaching the Confrontation stage doesn't mean you still can't get out of the attack. Just realize that the ABCs are progressive, so the earlier you can shut it down, the easier it is. Let's briefly explore these ABCs.

Psychological Self-Defense – Awareness:

While all three of the stories above are different, each one of them shows a failure of the first principle of Psychological Self-Defense—Awareness.

Awareness is your first line of defense in every situation. A lack of awareness means you're setting yourself up for a potentially dangerous confrontation.

What exactly is awareness?

Awareness means being attuned to your surroundings and your situations. It means using your senses—your sense of sight, hearing, and even smell—to observe the environment around you.

It means being aware of people and of what tends to happen in certain situations. It means being aware of things that don't fit, things that stand out from the norm.

Let's take the example of Kevin, the student. He's walking across a deserted campus at night all alone. He's completely unaware of his surroundings. His iPod drowns out his hearing, and he can't hear anyone approaching him. (Also, to a potential mugger, those white iPod earphones are a dead giveaway that there's a highly valuable iPod to be had.) He fixes his eyes downward and hunches over. He now can't see anyone approaching him.

He's not aware of his surroundings, which is obvious to any possible predator lurking around, hoping to catch a straggler at the end of exam week.

Kevin's may seem like an obvious example, but it gets a little more complex with Salma and Stacey.

These are just two normal girls enjoying a relaxing getaway in another country. How does the lack of awareness come into play here?

First of all, they're not aware (or don't realize) that different countries have different rules. (These are cultural boundaries that we'll talk about later.) What you can get away with in your hometown is not always what you can get away with in a completely different culture.

In some cultures, for example, two white, blonde, beautiful women that dress in tight clothes and short skirts are not only offensive to the people of that culture, but they are also prime targets for pimps, con artists, and sex traffickers.

There's another aspect of awareness here.

Salma had an instinct that warned her not to get into a car with Juan. She had legitimate doubts, but she pushed them aside. She didn't listen to her instinct or her doubts and let her friend persuade her into going.

Awareness doesn't just mean being aware of the outside world. It means being attuned to your inner world and instincts as well. Salma ignored her instincts, which in this case could have saved her.

Now let's talk about Chris. He missed several opportunities to use awareness to his advantage and avoid a fight.

First of all, Chris is at a bar drinking, and he's sitting down with two big, burly guys who are also drinking. He doesn't stop to think that:

#1: These guys are complete strangers; he really knows nothing about them.

#2: These guys are drinking. Drunk people have fewer inhibitions and can act in ways they wouldn't normally act.

#3: There are two of them and one of Chris. He's outnumbered.

The second thing he notices—but fails to act on—is the fact that they are leering at his girlfriend when she goes to the washroom.

Another clue Chris might have picked up on was the two guys acting like MMA fighters. Clearly these guys are brawlers, or at least think of themselves as such.

Finally, Chris is not aware of time or of the fact that most people have left the bar because it's near closing time. So there's nobody to help him or Tina when things go south.

By the time the guys started making lewd comments to Tina, it was already too late. Because of their lack of awareness, Chris and Tina got themselves into hot water.

In the first few chapters we're going to talk about this principle of awareness and start developing your awareness skills.

You're going to learn how to be aware of your environment and spot trouble before it starts. You'll also learn how to use to your God-given instincts to sense potential danger ahead of time.

We'll journey into the mind of a predator and learn how they select their victims, and what you can do to avoid being one of them. This is a level of awareness that most people never even know exists: Predators use very specific selection processes to target their victims.

Finally, we'll examine how to avoid the slow poisoning of emotional predators like sociopaths and narcissists that target your life. This will help you identify and avoid covert, psychological attacks.

Psychological Self-Defense – Body Language and Boundaries

The next level of self-defense after Awareness is the 'B' in your ABCs, which actually stands for two things—Body Language and Boundaries.

Reading body language is a powerful skill that very few people use today. However, it can give you endless information on whomever you are observing, including their real feelings (vs. what they are saying) and their hidden intentions towards you.

And it's not just other people's body language. You can use your own body language as well to send predators running the opposite way.

You actually use body language every day to send messages to people. We're going to uncover some tricks you can use to send the right messages—messages you want to send instead of messages that may be giving you results you don't want.

For example, when he hunched over and looked at the ground, Kevin unknowingly sent the message to his future mugger that he was a prime target. He looked small and fearful instead of powerful and confident.

By acting flirty and sexy—just as they acted at home—Stacey and Salma sent the wrong message. It may have been considered socially acceptable at home, but in another country it could easily have been misinterpreted.

You're also going to learn about a specific kind of body language—how to spot a liar. If someone is continually lying to you, it is an act of aggression towards you, even if it's not physical. You'll learn signs to look for to spot a pathological liar in this section of the book.

After body language, you're going to learn all about boundaries, both physical and psychological. Boundaries is a topic that doesn't get a lot of press these days, but it's a great tool that will help you know when someone is crossing the line so that you can head them off BEFORE they go further in their assault.

Establishing boundaries is also a simple, easy way to protect yourself from the everyday riffraff that comes sniffing around you, looking for a potential victim. Boundaries send an immediate message that you're not the right victim for them.

Boundaries are about your personal space. We each have boundaries, and we each have *the right* to have our own boundaries.

Nobody has the right to cross your boundaries without your permission, regardless of whether they've helped you out, bought you an expensive dinner, or hold a position of authority over you (e.g., your boss, a religious leader, a doctor, etc.).

Here's why boundary awareness is so crucial: Predators usually don't just attack you out of nowhere. Sometimes they do, but more often they come on slowly. And it often begins by testing your boundaries to see what you'll let them get away with.

They may cross a boundary to see what you do. If you let them get away with it, they may feel empowered to go further. And on and on it goes until you draw the line.

Unfortunately, if you let them go beyond a certain point, it may be too late. You want to recognize a boundary violation from the very beginning so that you can do something about it ASAP.

In the example with Chris and Tina above, the first boundary that was crossed was when Carl and Mike leered at Tina when she went to the restroom. Chris ignored that and gave them the benefit of the doubt because they were 'just being guys'.

They crossed the second boundary when they got a little too personal and started talking about Tina being hot. Then it escalated to talk about her being nude—a major boundary violation. If it hadn't been too late by that time, that should have been a red flag for both Tina and Chris to get out quick.

A boundary for you might be when you meet a guy for the first time on a blind date and he starts talking about sex in the first five minutes. Or maybe a coworker starts arguing with you and crosses the line of your personal space to get right up in your face.

There are lots of ways that predators test and cross our boundaries; we're going to learn how to identify them so that you can stop them and head off potential attacks.

Psychological Self-Defense – Confrontation

Finally, we get to the 'C' of the ABCs—the Confrontation.

Believe it or not, even if you get to the Confrontation stage, there are still things you can do to avoid a full-scale blowup. We're going to cover these things, including how to use powerful verbal and visual tactics to de-escalate a tense confrontation.

And if things do get to a red-alert state and turn physical? If all of your psychological self-defense skills fail and the crap hits the fan?

We're going to talk about that, too. You still have options. There are still things you can do to get out of the situation alive and with minimal damage.

So now that you have a brief overview of the ABCs, let's get started with the 'A'—Awareness.

Important Points:

◊ Psychological Self-Defense starts with your ABCs: Awareness, Body Language and Boundaries, and Confrontation

◊ The ABCs are progressive. You want to stop an attack at the earliest stage possible, which is the Awareness stage. If not, you can try to stop it at the Body language or Boundaries stage. If not, you can still try to avoid a physical attack at the Confrontation stage by using verbal and visual skills.

◊ Awareness means being both aware of your environment and being aware of yourself—your gut instincts.

◊ Body language means both reading other people's body language for hostile intentions and using your own body language to dissuade a possible predator.

◊ Boundaries are your personal borders or limits that are there to protect you; they can be physical, emotional, and mental. Everyone has the right to have their own boundaries.

◊ Predators will often violate your boundaries to see what you do. If you let them continue, it can be a signal for them to keep going and attack further.

◊ When you get to the Confrontation stage, you can still avoid an attack by using verbal and visual skills to de-escalate a situation.

Chapter 4 –
Avoid Dangers before They Start: How to Become an Awareness Super-Ninja

By Chuck O'Neill

"Most self-defense experts agree that nine out of ten dangers can be identified and avoided simply by learning how to look out for them."
— Lawrence A. Kane and Kris Wilder,
The Little Black Book of Violence

"Close your eyes," I tell them.

The room usually quiets down after a few nervous giggles.

"Now," I say, "think about where you are—the room that you're in and the people you're with. Take a moment and really think about it. In a few moments I'm going to ask you some questions. Pay attention to how many questions you can answer with complete certainty."

After a few moments I ask:

"How many people are in the room?"

"What color are the walls of this room?"

"Is there a clock?"

"Is there a fire alarm?"

"How many viable exits are there?"

"Are there double doors or single doors?"

"What color shirt is the person to your right wearing?"

"Is the person to your left wearing pants, jeans, or a skirt?"

"What kind of objects are on the table in front of you?"

"What is the energy of the person to your left? High energy? Mellow and calm?"

Then I tell them they can open their eyes and see how many questions they were able to answer correctly.

Most people are shocked at how few questions they actually get right. One, maybe two, three at most.

This is a great exercise to get people thinking about awareness. In fact, you can try it right now. Just keep your eyes closed or on the words in the book. Don't look around first! See how much you can actually recall about your current environment.

The truth is that most of us are trapped in our own worlds—in our relationship issues, in our problems, in our jobs, in our daydreams or goals.

We walk around with our noses stuck in our iPhones or Blackberries. Or we're focused on our notes or our laptop. We're so consumed with our busy lives that we fail to pay attention to what may be happening around us.

We're awake but not aware.

And, unfortunately, this can get us into trouble.

Being aware is the first key step in protecting yourself. Almost 80 percent of confrontations could be avoided or de-escalated if the victim had been practicing the skills of awareness.

What is awareness exactly?

Awareness is being cognizant of the circumstances and environment that you are currently in.

Now, being aware does not mean being paranoid. There's always a balance. Most of us are out of balance the other way—we're aware of very little. However, being paranoid about every little thing that moves around you, every place you go, is also out of balance the other way.

The key is to figure out which situations call for high-level awareness and which situations call for low-level awareness.

Four Main Levels of Awareness: Green, Yellow, Red, and Black

#1: Green Mode – Completely Unaware: When you're in green mode, you're pretty much completely unaware of what's going on around you. Maybe you're texting in a coffee shop or you're lounging at home reading a book. You might be studying in a library or completely mesmerized while playing the latest first-person shooter game at a friend's house.

Being in green mode isn't necessarily a bad thing. There are times we need to just relax and go 'green'. For example, you probably don't really need to be aware of your surroundings while reading a book at home. It's healthy to be able to unplug at times.

However, if you stay in green mode when you shouldn't be— say you're texting your friend in a bar where a loud argument breaks out between the couple beside you—that can be a problem.

#2: Yellow Mode – Aware and Cautious: When you're in yellow mode, you're aware of what's going on around you and watching for possible problem areas. You're cautious but still fairly relaxed.

You're not hyper-aware. But you're watching the situation develop around you with interest. You don't expect trouble; however, you also know that there's a small possibility it could develop.

For example, you might be in yellow mode when meeting with a potential new client at their office—a place you've never visited before in an unfamiliar area of town.

Another place you may be in yellow mode might be your favorite bar on a Friday night (where you know fights sometimes happen). Chances are nothing will happen, but when you throw a lot of drunk, horny people into the mix, it's always smart to be watchful.

#3: Red Mode – Hyper-Aware and Ready to Act: Red mode is hyper-aware mode; it's 'danger zone' mode. You're looking for trouble, and you think there's a fairly good chance it could occur.

Red mode is also action mode. In red mode you'll want to take steps as quickly as possible to remove yourself from the situation or get as far away from it as you can.

For example, you would switch from yellow to red mode in the bar example above if you noticed the guy next to you was arguing with his buddy, pumping his fist, and knocking over chairs and drinks.

You will immediately want to start thinking about how to get as far away from this situation as possible. You may want to leave the bar. You may want to go over to the far side of the room and watch. Either way, you'll want to take action if possible.

Another example of going into red mode is when you notice a stranger approaching your car, waiting for you to get out. Unless you're in a place where you're expecting this (like at a service station), this situation should be making you hyper-aware.

In that case, you may choose to lock your car doors and drive away to another parking spot.

By knowing about these first three levels of awareness, you can easily cycle among them and determine when to relax and when to take action. You also want to use these three modes in order to avoid ever getting into the fourth mode—the black mode.

#4: Black Mode – Shocked and Unable to Act: This is the last stage of awareness when facing a confrontation, and it's a level you don't want to get to. If you take action steps in the red mode, you can usually avoid ever getting into the black mode.

Black mode is basically game over. You're in the middle of the danger and you effectively shut down. You can't move. You can't think. Fear has taken over and adrenaline has basically shut down all areas of higher-level thought or action.

You don't want to get into this mode. However, just be aware that it can and will happen if you aren't monitoring the three other levels of awareness.

In his book *The Survivors Club*, Ben Sherwood talks about the theory of 10-80-10. In a crisis situation, 10 percent of people will take action in a relatively calm and rational state of mind. (These are often the people who do best in the crisis—the survivors.)

The majority of people (the 80 percent) will go into shock and disbelief, sometimes following what they see others do and sometimes doing nothing. This isn't necessarily fatal; you just need to recover from this shock quickly and take action (i.e., recover from the black mode).

Then there's the last 10 percent. These are the people who do the absolute worst thing. They freak out, lose control of themselves, and usually make the situation worse. These are the people that are in black mode and can't recover. Many times they don't survive the crisis.

Why Should You Know These Different Levels of Awareness?

You should know these different levels because they're a great tool you can use to see violence coming at you well before it happens. Most people who get into physical altercations tell me the same thing:

"It just happened. I didn't see it coming!" or

"It just came out of nowhere!"

But that's not entirely true.

The truth is they may have seen it coming if they'd been in orange or red mode. But because they were in green mode, they were completely unaware of what was going on around them. So they truly *didn't* see it coming.

> *"Most people who find themselves involved in violence think that they were just minding their own business and when they look up, suddenly this problem comes out of nowhere. It just seems like this at the time, though.* **There is virtually always some type of build-up**, *something they didn't see or didn't recognize the significance of until it became a problem."*
> *— Lawrence A. Kane and Kris Wilder,*
> *The Little Black Book of Violence [emphasis added]*

The Four Main Areas of Awareness:

There are four different areas where you can develop your awareness skills. Some experts put all of these under the blanket term 'situational awareness'. However, I wanted to break them out for you to help you get a better understanding of how to use them.

#1: Environmental Awareness

#2: People/Animal Awareness

#3: Energy Awareness

#4: Congruency Awareness

#1: Environmental Awareness: Environmental awareness means being aware of your physical location. For example, it might mean being aware that you're driving in a bad part of town. It might mean realizing that you're walking on a deserted side street instead of the main road to get to a bank machine. It may mean walking into a new client's home and making sure you know how many exits you have in case you need to leave in a hurry.

You don't have to be paranoid here, just observant of the area around you. For example, my wife is always much more aware when she is in underground parking lots versus when she is at home or at her favorite local Starbucks.

When she's in an underground parking lot, she's at the yellow mode of awareness—aware but not expecting anything bad to happen. However, if she notices that there aren't many people around and a large male stranger is approaching her, she shifts from yellow to red.

Whenever I did bodyguarding assignments for clients, I was hyper-aware of the situation (in red mode). I'd research the type of area (high end, white collar, industrial, etc.) my client was going to be in (commonly called 'advance work'), how many exits were in the building (including windows), where my client would be positioned relative to those around him or her, any possible hiding areas or hidden corners, etc.

This kind of situational awareness may be a bit much for you, but you get the idea.

In my Jamaican experience, I failed to be aware that my wife and I were heading into a bad part of town, a town where, because of our skin color and dress, we clearly did not fit in.

The next time you go into a potentially 'yellow' situation, try practicing environmental awareness. Ask yourself questions like:

- What is the area like?

- Have I been there before?

- How many exits are there?
- Will it be crowded or empty?
- Will I fit in with the crowd or will I stand out?
- If I had to get out of the situation fast, how could I do it?

Environmental Awareness:
How to Have a Safer, More Enjoyable Vacation

When travelling to new locations (for example on vacations or business trips), you can save yourself a lot of headaches and increase your personal safety by spending a few minutes doing what security experts call 'advance work'. Here are a few tips:

#1: Check your governmental travel advisory.

You can search them online with the phrase 'YOUR COUNTRY travel advisory for VISITING LOCATION'. You will get any security advisories, including areas to avoid. Canadians and Americans can check out the following sites:

CANADA: http://travel.gc.ca/

USA: http://travel.state.gov/

#2: You can also register your travel plans with the government site.

This way, if there is a national emergency, the local embassy will try and contact you. I also get the address and contact information for the local embassy. Then, if I lose my passport or end up in trouble with the authorities and need emergency assistance, I have that information on hand.

#3: Check out a couple of local papers online.

You can do this most of the time for free. I look at the crime section (this gives me an idea of where not to go), the political section (this gives me a sense of the stability of the country), and the social section (this gives me an idea of what is important to the local people).

By knowing these things, you can often converse with the locals (like your cab driver) and even get better service.

#4: If you're going to a country where the primary language is not one that you speak, learn some key phrases, such as:

"I need a doctor."

"I am a (your nationality here)."

"I have (chronic ailment such as diabetes, high blood pressure, etc.)."

"How much is it?"

"Hello, how are you?"

#5: Use an online map tool (e.g., Google Maps) and find out how far it is, approximately, from the airport to your hotel.

This way you can tell if your driver decides to take you on a 'tour of the island' versus taking you directly to your hotel. I usually allow for about 20 minutes extra in addition to what the map system shows because of traffic or construction. (So don't panic if it takes a little longer than you thought.)

#6: Research the cultural norms of where you're going.

Your travel agent may be able to help, but using the Internet you can usually find most of what you need to know online. Look for things like proper attire, prominent religion, and religious customs to popular social gestures.

#2: People/Animal Awareness: The second area of awareness is people. (It can also be potentially dangerous animals like dogs, as well.) Being aware of people can mean a lot of things.

It might mean noticing the man who's more interested in watching you at the grocery store than he is in picking out the cheapest toothpaste. It could mean noticing that the stranger on the plane next to you is asking a lot of personal questions and not telling you anything about himself in return. It can mean being aware of your coworker's depressed mood or their current life situation. (For example, are they losing their job? Do they have a wicked temper? Are they going through a divorce?)

We're going to talk a lot more in this book about being people-aware, including observing people's body language, reading their actions, and more. However, for now, you may just want to start practicing this skill and seeing what you come up with.

Ask yourself questions like:

◊ Who is near me right now?

◊ How close are they and is that 'normal'?

◊ What are they wearing and is it appropriate (for the weather or occasion)?

◊ Are they acting in a way that is 'normal' or appropriate for the current environment?

◊ (When dealing with people you know) Are they acting 'normal' or not?

Years ago, when I helped out in the Loss Prevention Department at a local department store, I found it much easier to identify shoplifters when I started to ask these two 'People Awareness' questions:

#1: "Are they acting 'normal'?" and

#2: "What are they wearing—and is that suited to the environment?"

#3: Energy Awareness: This basically involves being aware of the energy around you—and if it fits the environment. It can apply to both the situation and people. Think of this as the 'vibe' or 'atmosphere' of the place.

For example, you might be at an elegant restaurant that is usually subdued. But for some reason the energy has suddenly gone from subdued to tense and anxious. The energy has changed. Or maybe you work where the environment is usually cheerful and productive, but over the past week, it's started to grow negative, depressed, and slow.

I've had students tell me they knew when someone was about to hit them, simply from the energy change in their conversation.

When you become aware of sudden shifts in energy, be ready to move from yellow to red mode—and make a move. For example, if you're at a bar and the energy switches from laid back and slightly drunk to angry and hostile, get out of there.

If you find yourself in a group of friends and the energy suddenly switches from friendly to agitated—or even hostile—find an exit right away.

Start noticing the energy of different situations you go into this week. Observe the baseline energy of people and places. (The baseline is the normal level of energy.)

When something occurs that is out of the ordinary and not the baseline, it could be a warning that something is about to go down.

#4: Congruency Awareness: When I was a kid, I used to play games on those long road-trip vacations. One of them was called 'One of These Things Is Not like the Other'. It was basically two pictures: the main one and then a second one which would differ in some small way.

The guy in the picture might have six fingers instead of five. Or he might be wearing a helmet instead of a baseball cap. The whole point was to find the slight differences and circle them to find out what didn't match the main picture.

The fourth area of awareness is very similar to this game—being aware of what fits and what doesn't fit, or what's the norm and not the norm. This is also known as 'congruency' or 'incongruency'.

This could mean anything from noticing the girl in the heavy winter jacket in the middle of summer to the guy who seems nervous entering the office where he lost his job the day before.

When looking for things that don't fit, ask yourself this question:

"What stands out in this picture?"

It doesn't have to be extreme; it can even be subtle. But it's *key* to notice that it doesn't really fit the situation.

For example, let's say a stranger approaches you and asks for the time, but you notice he's wearing a watch. Does that fit the situation? Now, maybe he's just trying to pick you up. But then again, he may be trying to get close so that he can mug you.

Or how about a guy you've been dating for a while who still won't give you his home number? Does anything seem odd about this? He may be giving all sorts of excuses, but do they really add up to you?

Or what about the 20-year-old hottie who approaches you in a bar and practically begs you to take her home? If this happens to you every weekend, it isn't out of the norm. But if you've been happily married for 30 years and have never been hit on by this type of woman before, then something doesn't fit and you have to ask yourself why.

Here are some other examples of things that don't fit:

◊ Anyone who appears to be watching you in a store or other public environment

◊ Running into the same person in your usual spots over and over again

◊ Someone who changes their behavior based on your behavior (e.g., they stop walking when you stop walking, they change directions when you change directions, their plans change when your plans change)

◊ A car parked across from your house that doesn't belong to the neighbours or their friends—and the driver does not get out

◊ Somebody wearing clothes that don't fit with social standards and weather conditions

◊ Someone whose 'energy' doesn't fit their immediate environment

◊ A repairman or city worker who wants access to your home when you weren't given any written notice of the event

◊ A person you don't know showing sudden, intense interest in you

When you notice people or things that don't fit, it's not an automatic sign that something is horribly wrong. It's just a sign that more investigation is needed.

You'll want to take steps to investigate, ask more questions, and bring your awareness level into the red mode.

So those are some of the key areas of awareness. There is a fifth one we're going to cover in the next chapter: awareness of yourself. This involves trusting your instinct and tuning into situations that don't feel right, even if you can't quite reason it out logically.

However, before we move on to that, here's an example of how one of my students, Ken, used the skill of awareness to diffuse an attack.

Awareness in Action – Ken's Story:

Ken works as a manufacturing manager for a large, well-known company. He likes the job. But a few years ago, the company hit a rough patch. He had the unfortunate task of having to fire quite a few of his guys.

I'd been training Ken privately for a while, and we'd been discussing this skill of awareness. He came in one night and told me his story.

Ken, unfortunately, had to fire a man one morning who'd been at the company for 20 years. The man was a large, burly type who was understandably upset about losing his job. He'd been escorted out by security—along with the contents of his locker—around 10:00 a.m. that morning.

Ken worked all day and finished up around 6:00 p.m. As the manager, he was one of the last guys to leave every day. There were a few stragglers left in the plant, but there was nobody in the parking lot as he headed out to his car.

That's why it was so easy to notice the man he'd fired that morning, standing beside Ken's car waiting for him. Ken immediately knew he was facing a red mode situation. His awareness of the man skyrocketed.

He greeted the man calmly but positioned himself at a 45-degree angle to him. (Face-to-face contact can make an attacker feel even more aggressive.) He also made sure he kept five to six feet between the man and himself.

Then he listened as the man ranted. He had been at the company for over 20 years—they owed him something. He had a small daughter to support, etc. Ken listened sympathetically but all the while watched the man's body language and listened to his words.

The man repeatedly made a fist with his right hand and then released it as he talked (also known as 'fist pumping' in body language terms). He did this over and over again.

At the same time Ken noticed that the man's sentences had gone from long and fairly well thought out to short and blunt.

When the man's fist suddenly stopped pumping, Ken knew what was coming. He got ready for it.

The man lunged at him, aiming for his jaw. But because Ken had put so much space between them, he had time to step aside, grab the man's fist, and use his momentum to knock him on the ground. He then used his Wing Chun skills to take him down and land a knee in his back.

Ken's keen awareness skills in that situation saved him from a bloody nose, broken jaw, or worse.

Ken used the skills of awareness to do everything right in this situation.

First of all, he was aware that there were few people in the parking lot that night; his awareness level was on yellow already. Then when he saw a man—who should have left that morning and had waited around all day—his level went to red.

He identified that this was out of the ordinary—it didn't 'fit'. Nobody waits around at a job he was fired from that morning unless he has a serious axe to grind.

He used situational awareness to put at least five feet between himself and his adversary. He knew the man's situation was not conducive to a peaceful mindset (lost his job, had a daughter to support, felt the company owed him after 20 years of service, etc.). He also knew that this particular man had a reputation for being argumentative and sometimes physically hostile at the plant.

Furthermore, he had seen the man doing the fist pump, and when the man suddenly stopped pumping, he knew the man was preparing to strike.

He'd also listened to the man use long, detailed sentences (an indication of higher brain function) and gear down to short, one-syllable statements (an indication of lower brain functions kicking in, including the instinct to fight).

Ken is a great example of someone who used awareness to stop an attack.

Now, even if Ken didn't know Wing Chun (a form of Kung Fu) or any other martial arts, he could still have used awareness in this situation to protect himself. He could have seen the man waiting at his car when he stepped out of the building and simply walked back into the building and alerted security.

So this is a great real-life example of how one person used all four areas of awareness to diffuse an attack.

#1: He was aware of the environment (man who lost a job, empty parking lot).

#2: He was aware of the person (man who had a reputation as a fighter, man who was extremely upset and angry).

#3: He was aware of the energy. (At first it was high and angry, then it suddenly dropped as the man stopped fist pumping and gathered his courage to strike.)

#4: He was aware of what 'didn't fit' (incongruency—a man who waits around all day after being fired is not normal).

By continually being aware of the environment around you, the people, the energy and things that don't fit, you can cycle among the different modes of awareness and spot trouble coming before it starts.

And the more you practice, the more natural it will become until you hardly have to think about it.

You'll learn more about these areas of awareness throughout the book. However, there is one further area of awareness that is a fundamental self-protection tool—awareness of yourself and your gut instincts. That's what we'll cover in the next chapter.

Important Points:

◊ Most people are not aware of their environment, and this can make them easy targets for predators.

◊ Awareness is being cognizant or knowledgeable about your current circumstances.

◊ There are four main levels of awareness—green, yellow, red, and black. Cycle through these levels, depending on your situation, and always be ready to take something from yellow to red mode.

◊ Red mode is also action mode; be ready to take action to remove yourself from the situation when you hit red mode.

◊ Try to avoid black mode as it can cause a complete shutdown of higher brain function and the ability to act.

◊ There are four main areas of awareness:

1. Environmental Awareness

2. People Awareness

3. Energy Awareness

4. Congruency Awareness

◊ It's not hard to improve your awareness level. Practice being more aware of what's going on around you every day, and it will quickly become second nature to you.

Awareness Exercise:

You can do this exercise anywhere you are (where you can close your eyes). You can do this anytime you want. It will improve your awareness level and build your awareness skills.

#1: Close your eyes.

#2: Take a deep breath and focus on being in the present right now.

#3: Focus on your sense of hearing.

What do you hear? Do you hear anything unusual? Do you hear sounds that are normal to the environment? Are there any sounds you'd expect to hear but don't?

Is there somebody talking? What are they saying? Is this what you'd expect to hear from them?

#4: Now focus on your sense of smell.

What do you smell? Are there any smells that don't fit with the environment you're in?

#5: Now think back (without opening your eyes) to the room or environment that you're currently in.

What do you recall seeing? How many people were around you? What was their energy like? What were they doing?

Was there anything unusual about the room you are in? What color was the room? How many exits are there in that room? Is anyone behind you? Can you see the main door or are you turned away from the primary exit?

#6: Open your eyes and see how accurate you were. Try observing again, this time with your eyes open. Do you notice anything new? Could you have positioned yourself better so that it would easier for you to observe the situation around you?

Practice this on a regular basis and you'll start to develop your awareness skills to the level of a security pro.

Chapter 5 –
Listening to That Little Voice Inside: The Survival Skill We All Naturally Have

By Kate O'Neill

"Intuition is always learning, and though it may occasionally send a signal that turns out to be less than urgent, everything it communicates to you is meaningful." — Gavin DeBecker, The Gift of Fear

I was 10 years-old. His eyes burned through me with an intensity that cut like a knife through butter. That was the day my instincts saved my life.

I was walking home from school through the park and had just come over a hill, heading towards the street. I had been let out from school 15 minutes earlier than the other kids because I had a piano lesson. So I was hurrying towards Mrs. Black's house, worried that I might already be late.

Because it was mid-afternoon on a school day, there was nobody around in that small-town community. Everyone was either at school or at work. Nobody but me. Nobody but him.

I was rushing as fast as my little legs would take me towards the street I had to cross to get to Mrs. Black's house. That's when I saw the beaten-up brown sedan.

It had been driving at a regular pace as I came over the hill into view. Then it slowed. Then it stopped as I came closer to the road.

That's when I saw him.

Older. Late 30s, early 40s. Brown hair. Start of a beard. Disheveled.

And staring at me.

Staring intensely. Almost ravenous—the way I imagined a lion must look before he kills a gazelle.

My entire body went cold; the blood in my veins turned to ice. My heart raced like a runaway locomotive.

I suddenly had the overwhelming urge to turn around and run, run over the hill, through the park, and back to the school. Get away from this car—this man.

My instincts were warning me, screaming at me to get away. But my brain kicked in and started to fight back.

"You can't run," it said. "You'll look like an idiot. Maybe this guy just needs directions. Maybe he's having car trouble. And after all, he's an adult. You're supposed to listen to adults. What's he going to think if you turn and run away like a moron?"

"RUN!" my instinct screamed back. "RUN NOW!"

But I kept walking forward, listening to my logical brain. I did, however, hesitate slightly, which he noticed. He motioned me to come over to his car.

"RUN!"

"Don't be silly. You can't run. You're already going to be late for your piano lesson. And then Mrs. Black will be mad. And your Mom will be mad since she's paying a fortune for these lessons. You're being paranoid. And what are you going to tell them if you run back to school? That you ran from a CAR? How stupid will you look then?"

"RUN NOW! NOW!"

Instinct isn't always eloquent. But it's very powerful.

The man motioned me over again. I looked around. There was nobody in sight, no other cars, no adults in the park, no kids coming from school.

And that's when I made the decision to listen to my instincts.

I turned around and ran. I ran as if my life depended on it, as fast as my little 10-year-old legs could carry me, praying the entire time that he wouldn't follow.

I ran up the hill to the park, out of sight of the car, and stopped to catch my breath against a tree. After a few seconds, I peeked around the tree towards the road. He hadn't followed me, thank God.

The car was still there, but a second later it pulled away from the road and drove off. Guess he wasn't having car trouble after all.

I'll never know exactly what would have happened that day if I had approached the car. But I do know one thing: Listening to my instincts probably saved me from a very dangerous situation.

I know this as an adult. And to most of us who know about child predators, we can see this situation for exactly what it was.

But I was 10 years old at the time. I had been taught to respect my elders and do what they said—even if I didn't know them. Adults always knew best, I'd been told.

And it was the 80s. We didn't hear as much about these kinds of things back then. Oh, there was a little bit of it, but it wasn't as prevalent as it is now.

I had never been taught about child predators. I had nothing but my instincts to go on that day. Looking back, I'm eternally grateful that I listened to them.

In his wonderful book, *The Gift of Fear*, Gavin De Becker says that our gut instinct—this 'sixth sense' we all have is there to protect us. Contrary to popular belief, this instinct is not some spiritual, magical, ethereal thing that we get from a far-off mystical place.

This instinct is actually a warning system that picks up on a host of unconscious signs that our conscious brain may not register. Instinct puts these things together. And when they don't add up, instinct sets off our alarm bells to try and save us.

So while our conscious brain may not pick up on certain signs, our unconscious does. It then sounds the alarm to our instinct that something is off.

For example, as a fairly naive kid, I had no conscious realization of many things that were happening in that situation. I knew only that some guy had stopped his car and was motioning me over.

But my unconscious may have been registering a whole lot more that wasn't right about this situation. Things like:

◊ What would an older man want with a 10-year-old girl that he didn't know?

◊ Why was he all alone in a beaten-up old car?

◊ What was a grown man doing out in the middle of the day when most men are at work?

◊ Why was he driving around a school area?

◊ Why was he staring at me in a way I'd never seen any grown man look at me before?

◊ Why was he so unkempt and disheveled?

There could have been a host of other clues my unconscious picked up on as well; I'll probably never know them all.

But the main thing is that my instincts were telling me to run. And I listened to them despite the arguments from my conscious mind.

Listening to your own instincts is another side of building your awareness skills—the 'A' in your ABCs. It's more of an inner awareness that you can rely upon to warn you of impending danger.

Unfortunately, however, most of us don't listen to our instincts until it's too late.

We listen to our logical mind instead. We listen to the arguments—we don't want to offend someone or look stupid in a situation. We tell ourselves that we're just being paranoid, that this person who creeps us out is really a kind, harmless, caring person.

And we may end up paying the price for it.

For example, in my situation, I kept walking towards that car until I was about 20 feet away from it. It could have been too late by the time I gave in to my instincts and ran. That man could have easily gotten out of his car and outrun me.

Now, when I talk about instinctual fear, I'm not talking about irrational fear that makes you scared of every stranger, every encounter, or every little bump in the night. I'm talking about that inner knowing down in your gut that something isn't right.

Sometimes this feeling can be quite subtle—you just don't trust that new babysitter for some reason. Or a man at work just seems a bit 'slimy' to you. You can't put your finger on it, but the feeling is there.

Sometimes this feeling can be very strong and come on quickly. You suddenly get this urge to not get on that elevator. You suddenly feel a compulsion to make sure your child is all right when he's gone quiet in the next room.

Regardless of whether it's subtle or strong, it's important that you learn to listen to it. Become aware of it.

And become aware of the fact that your brain will try and talk you out of it. It will try to make you ignore your instincts.

Ultimately it's your choice whom you listen to.

Not all gut feelings about people are warnings about predators. It may just be that this person is a gossip and a user, so your instincts are warning you to stay away.

It may be that this person doesn't like you but is putting up a fake front. And your instincts are telling you something isn't quite right with them.

It might be that this person is lying because they're too embarrassed to tell you the truth. And it has nothing to do with you—it's just about them.

Regardless, your instincts pick up on a lot of unconscious signals, signals that can be used to help you avoid difficult and dangerous situations.

Your instincts can warn you about everything from a jealous friend that gossips about you behind your back to a boyfriend who comes on way too strong and eventually ends up stalking you.

How to Develop Awareness of Your Instincts

#1: Take Time to Listen to Them: Most of us live outward-oriented. We listen to our friends, our televisions, our political and religious leaders. We also live in a go-go-go world.

So we never actually take the time to quiet down, look inside, and ask ourselves where we're at or what we really feel about certain situations or people.

We need to slow down and start turning inward a little more. Ask yourself what YOU really think—not what you're told to think, not what your friends think—but what you really think.

Respect your own instincts. They are reliable and can be trusted.

#2: Stop Giving Everyone the Benefit of the Doubt: This may sound harsh. There are some people who deserve your mercy and there are others who don't. You have to decide this by first watching people and separating out the ones who deserve the benefit of the doubt and those who don't.

How do you do this? Watch people and listen to them.

What do they say on a regular basis? What do they do on a regular basis? What is their overall character like? Are they trustworthy? Are they kind?

One of my favorite quotes is from Maya Angelou who says, *"When someone shows you who they are, believe them the first time."*

Unfortunately though, we tend to assign people characteristics that we have. So if you're a nice person who generally doesn't gossip and somebody around you is constantly cutting others down, you might say, "Well, I'm sure they don't really mean it. Maybe they're just going through a rough time right now."

No. They're a gossip. They're showing you who they really are. And if they're willing to gossip TO you, they're going to gossip ABOUT you.

Believe them and save yourself some grief ahead of time.

Instead of giving everyone you meet the benefit of the doubt, practice observing their actions first. By doing this you will pick up on things, and your instincts about people will start to make more sense.

For example, years ago a friend of mine, Mary, was invited to a family dinner to meet her brother's new girlfriend, Karen.

Mary is very outgoing and bubbly. She takes a keen interest in people and is always asking them about their lives, their kids, their families, their jobs, and more.

When I asked her how the dinner went, she looked concerned.

"You know," she said, "Karen is pretty and all. I asked her a lot about her family and she answered all my questions, and I'm sure she's a nice person."

"But?" I could tell she was holding something back.

"You know, she never asked me one thing about myself. Not one question. No interest whatsoever." She shrugged after a second. "I'm sure she was just nervous—after all, it was the first time meeting the family."

"I wouldn't be so sure," I said. "It seems to me that if you're trying to make a good first impression, you would show some interest in the other person you're trying to impress. I'd be careful if I were you."

Mary laughed it off and forgot about it. She just figured she was being too judgmental.

As it turns out, Karen married Mary's brother and never did show much interest in Mary. Mary wasn't invited to the wedding. (It was held at a Bahamas resort, so only the parents and a few close friends were invited.)

When Karen got pregnant with her first child, she had two baby showers; Mary wasn't invited to either.

Eventually, Karen ended up having multiple affairs while married to Mary's brother and leaving her two young girls to be with her latest boyfriend, devastating Mary's brother and family.

When people show you who they are, believe them the first time.

That's not to say that every predator will give out selfish narcissistic signs like Karen did. Some of them will be über-charming. But the key is that something will still feel *off* to you.

For example, many famous cult leaders were known for their ability to charm people.

In her book *Captive Hearts, Captive Minds,* author Madeleine Landau describes them this way:

"Cult leaders have an outstanding ability to charm and win over followers. They beguile and seduce. They enter a room and garner all the attention. They command the utmost respect and obedience."

Hitler was charming. Charles Mason was charming. The key, however, is to look at their actions—do they fit with their words?

Oftentimes when they do not, your instincts have already registered that something is off. Your instincts will be trying to warn you.

I once visited a church where the pastor was a well-known, charismatic leader. He was attractive, persuasive, and übercharming. When he spoke, he could get you so emotionally riled up you felt like you'd just sat through a World Series game and your team won.

But there was something off. I noticed that at several points during his sermon he took several Biblical Scriptures out of context and twisted them to fit his message—what he wanted to say instead of what was actually meant by the context.

The first time, I let it go. The second time, I started to get worried. By the third and fourth times, I was just plain uncomfortable.

Anyone can make the Bible say whatever they want if they take certain Scriptures out of their context. And the fact that a well-known religious leader—who should have known better—was doing so unnerved me. His actions weren't matching up with his words or image.

Funny enough, when we got into the car, Chuck mentioned that he had noticed the same thing—he'd noticed the exact four times the pastor had twisted Scripture that I'd noticed. He, too, was uncomfortable with this leader's sermon. His instincts—like mine—were sounding alarm bells about this man.

Several years later, we heard that this mega-church was now in shambles. It had split apart because of this man's tyrannical rule and controlling behavior behind the scenes that had gone on for years.

Don't always rush to give people the benefit of the doubt. Watch them first and trust your instincts. They will show you who they are over time.

By doing this you can also identify 'safe' people, people who are trustworthy, caring, and honest and who sincerely care about you.

I've used this principle to find some of the most amazing people that I'm privileged to call my friends—people who show genuine caring, thoughtfulness, and kindness. These people are the true treasures in life—and my life is all the better for having them in it.

I also use this principle to identify unsafe people, people who are narcissistic, selfish, self-involved and dishonest. And I take steps to keep them out of my life. It's just a lot less stressful that way—you sleep better at night.

By observing people and believing what they show you the first or second time they're around you, you can save yourself a lot of potential pain, drama, and emotional strife.

Important Points:

- ◊ Your instincts are there to protect you. Listen to them.

- ◊ Your instincts are a collection of signals picked up by both your unconscious and conscious minds. When something doesn't fit, your instinct 'alarm bell' goes off to warn you.

- ◊ Don't let your mind always rule your decisions, especially when your instincts are ringing alarm bells that go against your mind. It might warrant further investigation.

- ◊ Don't be afraid to look stupid or silly by listening to your instincts. Better to be safe and alive than to look cool but get attacked.

- ◊ Practice listening to your instincts by slowing down and looking inward occasionally.

- ◊ Don't automatically give everyone the benefit of the doubt.

- ◊ People show you who they really are by what they repeatedly do. Listen to them.

- ◊ Pay attention to people's actions, not how charming, charismatic, or good-looking they are. Ask yourself if what they do matches what they say.

Awareness Exercise:

#1: Recall a time in your life when you didn't listen to your instincts and something bad may have happened as a result (e.g., with an important work project, a boyfriend/girlfriend, a dangerous situation).

Do you recall getting any initial clues that something was off?

In what way were your instincts warning you?

How did your brain convince you to ignore your instincts?

If you had listened to your instincts in that situation, do you think things would have turned out differently?

What do you wish you'd done in that situation?

What's the main thing you can learn from that experience that will help you in the future?

#2: Recall a time in your life when you *did* listen to your instincts. What happened as a result?

What was the situation?

What was the deciding factor that made you trust your instincts?

Were you tempted to ignore your instincts? Why?

Were you ultimately satisfied with the outcome of the situation?

What's the #1 thing that you can take away from that experience?

Chapter 6 –
The Predator Interview: The Interview You DON'T Want to Pass

By Chuck O'Neill

> *"...before a bad guy tees off on you, he will evaluate his odds of success. This evaluation is often called an 'interview'... Passing means that you appear to be an easy target. To the other guy, you've got a giant 'V' for victim stamped on your forehead."*
> — Lawrence A. Kane and Kris Wilder,
> The Little Black Book of Violence

Almost every criminal or predator conducts what security experts call 'The Interview'. This is where they decide if you're going to be their next victim or not. You see, predators don't just attack anyone out of the blue. There is a specific selection process.

And to understand the interview, you have to understand the criminal mindset behind it. You have to understand what a predator fears:

He fears getting caught.

Even if he's the worst of the worst psychopathic criminals, he doesn't want to get caught and have to pay for his actions. So, logically, he wants to select the right victim that won't get him caught, exposed, or in trouble with the law. He wants an easy mark—physically, psychologically, or both.

So he 'interviews' you to see if you fit his criteria. He assesses whether or not you're going to fight back, whether you'll stand up to him, whether you're aware of your surroundings, or whether you'll be compliant and let him do whatever he wants.

(Note: I'm using the male gender here for the sake of simplicity; however, the predator could just as easily be a 'she'.)

Many women and even men who don't have a lot of experience in the security field have never even heard of the *interview*. But it's very real, and if you know how to fail the interview, you can send a predator on his way, looking for another victim.

"The criminal's process of victim selection, which I call 'the interview', is similar to a shark's circling potential prey. The predatory criminal of every variety is looking for someone, a vulnerable someone who will allow him to be in control, and just as he constantly gives signals, so does he read them."
— Gavin DeBecker, The Gift of Fear

There are many different types of interviews that we'll cover later in this chapter. But to help give you an idea of how this process works, let's go over a few examples.

Cheryl's Interview:

Cheryl was just starting to put away the MLS listing sheets when the man knocked at the screen door and let himself in. Tall, well-dressed, black wavy hair, and unusually good-looking, he caught her by surprise.

It had been a slow day for an open house, only a few potential buyers. And none had been as good-looking as this one.

"Hello there! I know I'm a bit late—do you mind? I was in the neighbourhood visiting some friends and saw your sign. My wife loves this area—great for kids. I was wondering if I could look around?"

Cheryl hesitated. Sure he was well dressed and seemed friendly enough, but she didn't know this man. And the open house was essentially over.

Still, a potential sale might be at stake. And if he was looking to buy a home and didn't have an agent already...

"Sure, go ahead." She gave in, motioning around her. "Look around and let me know if you have any questions."

"Thanks." He flashed her a mega-watt smile. "I know it's annoying for you agents when someone wanders in at the last minute. But I promise I won't be too long. Have you had many people come by today?"

Cheryl stacked up the unused MLS listing sheets but saved one out of the pile for him.

"A few. Not as many as I'd like, obviously."

The man laughed and wandered into the front living room area.

"Never is, I guess. My ex-girlfriend was a real estate agent for a few years, so I know the drill. Have you been an agent long?"

Cheryl crossed the kitchen to the living room to hand him the MLS listing sheet.

"Yes, quite a while actually."

The man took the sheet, brushing his hand against hers in the process.

"Thanks. I guess that means you're a pro then. How does your husband feel about you being an agent—no weekends off and all?"

"Oh, I get a few here and there." Cheryl didn't turn her back on him but waited until he'd wandered into the attached dining room before heading back to the kitchen. After a few minutes, the handsome stranger wandered into the kitchen and continued talking casually to her.

"I guess he just goes off and plays golf with his buddies, eh? That's what I'd do if my wife were busy all weekend."

Cheryl turned and faced him squarely. Keeping her voice polite but firm, she corrected him.

"Actually, he helps me clean up after every open house. In fact he should be here in about two minutes. What kind of house did you say you were looking for again?"

The man's smile faltered just slightly but then quickly recovered. He gestured into the air.

"Oh, something like this. It's not a bad little house."

She narrowed her eyes and pinned him with her gaze.

"And how many kids do you have?"

"Sorry?"

"You said your wife likes the area because of the schools. I assume you have kids," Cheryl pressed.

The man laughed and pasted a sheepish grin on his face. "Not yet—but soon I think. My wife wants kids soon."

"That's great. By the way, the owners of the home should be back any moment. So if you want to take a look upstairs, you'd better get to it."

She didn't care at this point if she sounded rude. This man was not what he appeared to be, and she wanted to make it plain that she wasn't amused by his fake charm or slimy come-ons. Her heart was pounding and she prayed the man was buying her story about her husband coming soon.

With another quick look around, the man moved back towards the door.

"No, that's all right. I've seen enough. I'll talk to my wife about the house and we'll call you if we're interested."

As he walked out the door without looking back, Cheryl smiled in relief and sank back against the kitchen table.

"Sure you will."

Cheryl failed the interview.

Kyle's Interview:

Kyle was knocking back a few drinks at his local pub with his girlfriend, Julie, and a few of her friends. Some of his buddies had cancelled at the last minute, so he was the only guy at their table. He felt a little like 'The Bachelor' and was currently enjoying the jealous glances of the guys at the next table.

Julie's friends were doing what they always did every weekend—dancing, flirting, picking up. At one point there were just Kyle and Julie left sitting at their table. They were the designated drink and purse-watchers.

"Was it something I said?" Kyle joked, with a sweeping gesture around their empty table. Julie laughed, shifting in her seat, pulling her chair in to let people pass their crowded table.

She apparently hadn't moved in close enough, however. A second later a large, burly drunk shoved her against the table in his efforts to get by.

Kyle blurted out, "Hey, WATCH it buddy."

The muscleman turned and eyed Kyle with his red, glazed eyes. "Watch WHAT? What're you gonna do about it?"

Kyle tried to use a calm voice as he shrugged it off. "Nothing man, just watch where you're going. You nearly crushed her."

But Mr. Muscles took that as a challenge. "I'll damn well go where I please, you pussy."

He looked Kyle over, sizing him up and taking in the lack of male friends at the table. Mr. Muscle, on the other hand, had three friends following behind him like obedient puppies. They were all now watching the exchange with interest.

"Just watch it—that's all I'm saying." Kyle shrugged.

"Trying to look cool, huh?" The bully challenged. "I think it's time YOU learned to respect who you're talkin' to."

The guy moved in closer to Kyle.

Raising his hands up and showing his palms, Kyle tried to placate his opponent again.

"Hey listen, we don't want any trouble. Just forget about it, okay?"

Steroid-boy smiled and started to roll his sleeves up.

"If you didn't want trouble, you shouldn't have opened your filthy mouth. Now you're going to pay for it."

Seeing the anticipation in the man's glassy eyes, Kyle knew exactly where this was going. The guy was double his size; he was probably going to get his ass kicked.

Oh well, here goes nothing, Kyle thought. He'd been taking martial arts classes for only a month. There was no way he could take a guy this size, but he did know the proper fighting stance. Maybe he could convince the guy he really knew how to fight.

Standing up slowly, Kyle drew himself up to his full height. He broadened his shoulders and tried to take up as much physical space as possible. Drawing back into his fighting stance, he gave the guy his most aggressive stare-down.

"Okay, if that's the way you want it." He motioned the guy forward. "Come and get me asshole. We'll see how long you last."

Mr. Muscles hesitated. He looked over Kyle's stance and seemed confused by the sudden intensity rolling off Kyle's body. Kyle could practically see the wheels turning as he tried to put it together.

"C'mon buddy," Kyle challenged in a low voice. "Everyone here knows you started this. Take the first shot."

Finally, after a few seconds, steroid-boy shook his head and knocked a chair over with his fist.

"Ahh, you're not worth it you little *&$%." He spit on Kyle's table before stumbling off to the bar.

Kyle failed his interview as well.

How to Fail an Interview

When looking for a victim, predators want things easy. They want to find someone who won't give them a hard time.

Just like a lion hunting gazelle, they don't want to work to take down the strongest gazelle in the herd. That's way too much trouble. They'll go for the easy kill—the weaker, slower gazelle.

That's why they interview you, just like a job applicant. They're looking for signs that you'll fit their requirement of an easy, pliable victim.

What are some ways they interview you?

◊ They may watch you from across the street five minutes before they mug you.

◊ They may observe you for a few weeks before they stage a 'meeting' as you're entering your apartment.

◊ They may strike up a conversation at the hotel bar and casually ask you if you're in town alone on business or meeting some work colleagues.

◊ They may approach you in the parking lot and ask you for directions to see how you respond.

◊ They may appear to be your friend at the local bar where you hang out together, where they subtly probe you about your personal life, job, financial situation, family, etc.

- ◊ They may test your boundaries as you're working with them in a client relationship, pushing ever further to see how far you'll let them go.

- ◊ They may stop you on the street with a sob story about being mugged and ask you to help them with spare change, a cell phone, a ride to somewhere, etc.

- ◊ They may make lewd comments on a first date to see how you respond.

There are many different ways you can be interviewed.

In the example above, the man appearing at Cheryl's open house was, in fact, a predator. He had watched her set up her sign and observed that, at the end of the day, she was alone in the house.

He'd wandered in at the last minute and tested her boundaries to see if she would let him look around after the official open house hours were over. He was counting on the fact that agents usually salivate at the thought of a potential new client or a sale.

His charming smile and high-end clothing had been used purposely to make her feel comfortable and at ease and to let him in when she might not have done so for a poorly dressed stranger.

He'd told her about his ex-girlfriend being an agent to establish common ground. It was also to put her at ease with him, so she'd be more willing to open up.

He'd asked her if she'd had many people come through to assess whether there was a lot of interest in the house—and whether there might be more people dropping by at the last minute to interrupt him.

He'd asked her if she'd been an agent long, both to establish rapport with her and to assess whether she knew the potential dangers of open houses hosted by lone female agents. He was looking for a new, naive agent, and Cheryl's answer about her years of experience didn't please him.

He'd asked about her husband, a presumptive question to find out if there was indeed a strong male presence in her life and if he might be coming by anytime soon.

When Cheryl had smartly advised him that her husband was on his way and the clients were due back any minute, he figured there were too many risks in making Cheryl his next victim. So he moved on.

What he hadn't known was that Cheryl's real estate agency regularly hosted talks on personal protection and how to be safe—especially as a female agent.

She had seen this man coming and recognized the signs.

Now, we could probably say that Cheryl should not have let him come in at the start, and perhaps that's true. However, Cheryl still didn't know much about this man. He could have been totally innocent—and a potential sale.

But she did watch him. And when things didn't add up, she purposely gave him signs that told him she was not going to be an easy victim.

She told him she was an experienced agent. She took control of the conversation and forced him to answer her questions about what kinds of houses he was looking for. She didn't turn her back to finish tidying up but faced him down with strong, confident body language.

And she told him that her husband was on his way (even though he wasn't).

She failed the interview, and the man went away in search of easier prey.

Now, the example with Kyle is a bit different. When it comes to guys vs. guys, you always have to deal with the male ego.

Sometimes you can avoid a confrontation by acting submissive and letting the other guy look like the alpha male. If he's a normal guy and just being a jackass (the everyday dumbass attacker from chapter two), this can often work as he doesn't really want trouble either. He just wants to look like the head dog over you. And if you let him do this, he'll move on, confrontation avoided.

This is what Kyle tried to do at the beginning when he tried to calm his burly challenger down.

However, this doesn't always work. And in the case of an especially aggressive predator, it can be an invitation to attack. They may see submission as an indicator of weakness, and you start looking like a prime target.

So in this case, Kyle did the smart thing—he changed tactics and confronted the bully. He used his body language to try and appear larger and more powerful than he really was. He assumed a fighting stance and acted like he was ready to use his mad Kung-Fu skills on his attacker.

His words then gave his adversary the idea that he was much more skilled than he actually was. And his intense, confrontational stare gave an air of confidence in his fighting ability. In Mr. Muscles's mind, this planted doubts.

Should he attack Kyle? What if Kyle was the next Bruce Lee? What if he was some black belt ninja that could kill him with a single strike?

Suddenly, Kyle didn't look like an easy target anymore. Suddenly, Kyle was looking like more trouble than he was worth.

Kyle failed the interview, and Mr. Muscles moved on to prey on a weaker adversary.

> "... even the simplest street crime is preceded by a victim selection process that follows some protocol .... Some aspects of victim selection (being the right appearance or 'type', for example) are generally outside the victim's influence, but those that involve making oneself available to a criminal, such as accessibility, setting and circumstance ... are determinable."
> — Gavin DeBecker, *The Gift of Fear*

The Four Different Types of Interviews

There are several different styles of interviews, depending on the predator's goals and intended actions. Here are a few of them:

#1: The Standard Interview: This is a common type of interview where a stranger approaches you on the street and asks you for something. You may be getting out of (or into) your car. You may be getting on the subway. You may be in a fairly deserted area off the main street getting money from a bank machine.

They may ask you for change, for the time, for directions, anything to distract you.

They're watching for a few things like:

- ◊ How you react. For example, do you give in to their request and try to help them or do you give them a firm 'No'.
- ◊ Are you aware of your surroundings? Or do you seem thrown off and disoriented by their question?
- ◊ Do you allow them to get close to you, or do you tell them to stop where they are and not come any closer?
- ◊ Do you maneuver yourself into a safe position with your back close to the wall or the car so that you can't get hit from behind?

In order to 'fail' your interview, make sure you are alert to your surroundings. Never let them get within five feet. (A woman may prefer six or seven feet.)

Look them straight in the eye and tell them 'No'. Or, if you can, avoid them (by not getting out of your car, driving away, walking into a store and talking to the owner, etc.)

#2: The Fast and Furious Interview: This is when an attacker comes at you from out of nowhere. The idea is that you'll be too shocked and disoriented to fight back.

They may have been hiding behind a car in the parking garage or behind some bushes on the street. They may have been hidden in the shadows of the alley as you passed by.

These interviews happen fast—there's no talking process involved.

But there is a type of interview process going on here—they watch you first.

They make their assessment, not by talking to you, but by looking you over. They may be judging your clothing choices, your body language, or even your shoes (e.g., "Can she run in those heels?").

They may be looking to see if you're aware of your surroundings or if you're lost in your own little world and won't notice their approach.

By walking confidently and looking like you're aware of your situation, you may manage to avoid an attack in this way. (Don't worry; you can still wear nice shoes.)

But sometimes this isn't enough and they attack. What can you do then?

Keep the goal in mind here: You still want to make them think you're going to be more trouble than it's worth. So you want to communicate this in any way possible.

Scream, threaten, swear, use aggressive body language, and if the situation warrants it, punch, kick, bite, elbow, knee—basically fight like hell.

It doesn't matter if you can't throw a punch to save your life. The main goal is to make them think that they picked the wrong target and that if they continue the attack, you're going to be a giant pain in the ass.

They may just reassess their choice, let you go, and move on to find an easier victim.

Side note: This does not mean you should stop your aggressive tactics until the attacker rests or backs off for a moment.

If you stop your attack midway, the attacker may intensify his assault to 'teach you a lesson' or 'put you in your place'. You have to keep going until the attacker stops his aggression towards you and has moved on.

#3: The Temperature-Rising Interview: This is an interview that starts out as a peaceful—and by all accounts normal—exchange. But then it quickly escalates into something else.

For example, the interview above with Cheryl, the real estate agent, was a temperature-rising interview. The man started out as a seemingly normal person crossing one innocent boundary (asking her to let him in after hours). He then proceeded to ask more personal questions, questions that a total stranger should not have been asking.

If Cheryl had been naive about these kinds of situations, she may have continued to let him cross the line, giving out the information he wanted. She may have let it slip that her husband was nowhere in the neighbourhood but was, in fact, away on a business trip.

She may have been flattered at this handsome man's obvious interest in her and agreed—as he was hoping—to show him upstairs to the bedrooms. From there, the interview would have escalated, and he would have attacked.

Another example might be a man who strikes up a conversation with a woman on an airplane. Through friendly back and forth questions, he manages to learn that she is on a business trip to Chicago on her own. She has no husband or boyfriend and will not be meeting anyone at the airport.

This interview can quickly escalate with a little more flirting and then an invitation to share a cab ride or even meet for dinner later on.

That's not to say that every time a woman gets hit on, the guy is a predator. There are a lot of perfectly acceptable guys that are just looking to score with a pretty girl this way.

The key is to look for what doesn't fit—what isn't normal. For example, Cheryl noticed that the man wasn't acting like a typical home buyer: He showed up late and he wasn't with anyone (most open house visitors are couples). He wasn't asking the usual questions about the house. He didn't ask for an information sheet; she had to give him one.

His answers were vague, and he was asking her much-too-personal questions. He was clearly probing her for information about her husband or a male influence in her life. And when she asked him if he had kids, he was clearly thrown off guard, which was unusual since he'd mentioned the schools in the neighbourhood earlier.

Too many things were not adding up, and since Cheryl had years of experience, she quickly knew the man wasn't a normal home buyer.

#4: The Extended Interview: This is an interview that takes place over time. The predator is watching you, talking to you, maybe even trying to start a friendship with you, all to assess your weaknesses, your character, your assets and your strengths.

A predator planning to con you in a business deal would do an extended interview. Some cases of stalking also fall into this category as well.

What should you do? Well, it always depends on the situation. But the main thing here is to use your awareness and listen to your instincts, which may tell you that something isn't right. Perhaps this person is just a little too good to be true; they almost don't seem human. Maybe they're trying to get too personal too fast.

They may be too pushy; they may manipulate you into doing things you didn't want to do. Or maybe they clearly don't listen to you when you say 'No'.

The good news with this kind of extended interview is that you have time. You can get away from the person or the situation if your instincts are telling you that something isn't right.

Look into their claims—are they legitimate? Do some research and see if what they're telling you is true. (You can learn a lot with a simple Internet search these days.)

If, for example, they claim to work somewhere, call the place and verify that they work there. If they make claims about their achievements (for example, they set a record for X, Y, or Z), check to see if this is correct.

Check the facts, especially if something is warning you not to trust this person.

And if you do find out they're not what they seem, the number one rule is this: Do Not Engage. They may try to bait you or use fear, guilt, or intimidation to keep you in contact with them, especially once they realize you've caught on to their game.

But resist the urge. Avoid all contact with them if possible. The best response in this situation is no response. They'll lose interest when they realize they can't push your buttons and hopefully move on to easier prey.

If they do persist, you should contact your local law enforcement to get some advice (which may include restraining orders, formal charges, etc.) You'll also want to inform a close friend or family member of the situation. This way you have witnesses if needed.

So those are four of the most common types of interviews and some tips to identify and deal with them.

Almost every predator goes through this process to find his (or her) next victim. The key to protecting yourself is to understand they are looking for an easy mark. Figure out how to make yourself look like the most difficult mark they've ever interviewed—and they'll most likely move on.

In the next chapter we'll talk some more about how to do this by understanding the psychology of your attacker. Let's go inside the mind of a predator and see how we can beat him.

Important Points:

◊ Almost every predator will conduct an 'interview' before attacking you to see if you're a good candidate to be their next victim.

◊ There are several different types of interviews, including:

#1: The Standard Interview – A stranger approaches to ask you some questions and see how you'll react.

#2: The Fast and Furious Interview – A stranger watches you and jumps you, giving you little time to react.

#3: The Temperature-Rising Interview – The interview starts out friendly in a seemingly normal situation but quickly escalates into an attack.

#4: The Extended Interview – The predator watches you over time to gauge your strengths, weaknesses, schedules, habits, and more.

◊ One of the best ways to fail an interview is to be able to identify when it's happening to you. From there, your goal is to convince your interviewer that you would not be a good victim—you're too strong, too much trouble to deal with, will put up too much of a fight, etc.

Awareness Exercise – The Interview:

#1: Put yourself into the role of a predator (only if you are comfortable with this role-playing exercise). Go to a mall or another high-traffic area. Try to pick out the one person who would be the easiest to attack.

Why did you choose them?

Are they displaying certain body language traits? Is it because they're wearing certain clothes?

Is it because they are texting or otherwise unaware of what's going on around them?

Do they have a certain energy about them?

Are you unknowingly doing these same things? How can you change this?

#2: Have you ever been interviewed? Think back to any run-ins with predators you may have had (or avoided) in the past.

Was there an interview process? What kind of interview was it (Standard, Fast and Furious, Temperature-Rising, Extended)?

What signals did you send? What signals did you wish you'd sent?

What signals could you practice sending in the future?

Chapter 7 –
They Don't Think Like You – Understanding the Mindset of a Predator

By Chuck O'Neill

> *"MRI scans of human beings' brains show a positive activity in the limbic (emotional) region when the subjects are shown highly disturbing images. When the same test is carried out on a psychopath, there is no activity registering in the limbic region. Psychopaths have no ability to feel empathy. The machinery is not there inside of the brain of a psychopath."*
> — Rik Atherton, *Self Defense Against the Psychopath: Essential Reading for Everyone*

Part of successfully avoiding becoming the next victim of a predator is in understanding one key concept:

Predators don't think like you.

Therefore, they won't play by the same rules that you do. You cannot trust or assume that they will do what you would do in a given situation.

Now, we're not talking in this chapter about the everyday dumbass predator from chapter two who wanders into a bad situation. We're talking about the really serious predators—the sociopaths, psychopaths, criminals, narcissists, and even the desperate, physically driven attackers.

I want you to understand that there are people out there for whom you cannot show mercy—people who will never back off once they've targeted you. So you must take steps to understand how they think and protect yourself.

And these predators think completely differently than you do.

To give you a taste of just how different predators think, here's a small sampling of quotes from famous sociopaths and criminals around the world:

"I've never killed anyone! I don't need to kill anyone! I THINK it! I have it HERE! [Pointing to his temple.] I don't need to live in this physical realm ..." — Charles Manson

When a judge asked Peter Kurten, a German serial killer, if he had a conscience, Kurten replied:

"I have none. Never have I felt any misgiving in my soul; never did I think to myself that what I did was bad, even though human society condemns it.

My blood and the blood of my victims will be on the heads of my torturers. There must be a Higher Being who gave in the first place the first vital spark to life.

That Higher Being would deem my actions good since I revenged injustice. The punishments I have suffered have destroyed all my feelings as a human being. That was why I had no pity for my victims."

"I don't feel guilty for anything. I feel sorry for people who feel guilt."
— Ted Bundy, serial killer

Question: "What do you think when you see a pretty girl walking down the street?"
Answer: "One side of me says, 'I'd like to talk to her, date her.' The other side of me says 'I wonder how her head would look like on a stick?'"
— Ed Kemper, serial killer

> "I don't even know if I have the capacity for normal emotions or not because I haven't cried for a long time. You just stifle them for so long that maybe you lose them, partially at least. I don't know."
> – Jeffrey Dahmer, serial killer

> "It wasn't as dark and scary as it sounds. I had a lot of fun .... Killing somebody's a funny experience."
> — Albert DeSalvo, a.k.a. the Boston Strangler

With that brief insight into the minds of some of the world's worst psychopaths and criminals, do you see why it's important to understand that they're not like you?

Do you see why, if you ever get in a situation where you are targeted, you can't be nice and hope for the best?

This is especially crucial for women, who are taught from the womb to be polite and submissive. But if someone is coming after you, being polite could get you killed.

When you understand that, you'll start to understand that it's okay to be mean, to be rude, and to fight like hell if the situation calls for it. I want you to have the attitude that says: "If you're going to come after me, buddy, it's going to be the worst experience of your life!"

Again, this is not to make your paranoid or to scare you. However, we have to look at reality here.

Martha Stout estimates in her book *The Sociopath Next Door* that nearly **1 in 25 people are sociopaths,** and that doesn't include other kinds of emotionally disturbed people like narcissists or just your everyday, run-of-the-mill criminal.

When I was taking my bodyguarding training, one of the top security experts in the U.S. informed us that at any one time, in any neighbourhood in North America, about 5 percent of the population could be classified as EDPs—Emotionally Disturbed People. This can include sociopaths, narcissists, criminals, personality disordered individuals, people with serious mental disorders, etc.

While these people are not the norm, chances are high that you'll come across several of them in your lifetime. So you need to understand how they think. As Sun Tzu said, *"Know Your Enemy."*

In the moment or time frame that these people are coming after you, they are not thinking like you would. While you may react in the normal, socially accepted way to events, they may not. For example:

- ◊ While you mean it when you make a promise, they will make a promise and break it without a drop of remorse.
- ◊ While you react to somebody asking for mercy—and grant them that mercy—a predator will grant you no mercy.
- ◊ While you may think that showing a predator love and kindness will win them over (because it would win you over), they will see it as weakness and see you as an easy mark.
- ◊ While you would cringe at the thought of playing mind games with someone and making them doubt themselves to the point of self-loathing, a predator will see this as a fun game.

It can be hard to wrap your mind around this concept. And it does take some time to accept. But if you ever get into a physical confrontation, the one thing I want you to remember is that you can't trust a predator to think like you'd think or act like you'd act.

Let's talk about someone who has crossed the line and is coming after you physically. If they're trying to kidnap you, rape you, steal from you, or beat you up, they've already shown that they're willing to cross the boundaries of polite social conventions.

So at that point, all bets are off. They aren't going to adhere to other boundaries of polite social conventions either, like keeping their word:

"I promise I'll let you go after you let me do this."

"I promise I won't hurt you if you just get in the car with me."

"Just give me your wallet and I'll go."

They're not going to tell you the truth. They're not going to listen to your appeals for mercy or your appeals to their conscience. (They have none.)

They're not going to be guilt-stricken that they are harming you and go away.

If you want to fight them you have to know this and react accordingly. You have to realize that all bets are off, and if you're going to survive, you can't rely on their goodness, kindness, humanity, guilt, or honesty. You have to fight like hell and rely on yourself in this situation.

The Emotional Predator

We've talked a lot about physical attackers. But the predator mindset doesn't always translate into physical violence. It can also translate into more subtle attacks, designed to hurt you in non-physical ways. It could be:

- ◊ A work colleague who destroys your reputation at the office by planting tasty bits of gossip about you over time.

- ◊ A jealous friend who gives you subtle digs about your weight, your clothing choices, or your hairstyle, slowly destroying your confidence.

- ◊ An attractive young woman at the office who seems open to an affair only to take you for everything you're worth when she's finally got you.

In the movie *White Oleander*, Michelle Pfeiffer plays Ingrid, a sadistic, narcissistic mother who murders her boyfriend and goes to jail, leaving her teenage daughter, Astrid, at the mercy of the system, getting passed around to different foster homes.

After several rough starts, Astrid finally goes to stay with a kind, loving woman named Claire. Claire encourages Astrid and adds some much-needed stability to her life. However, the jealous Ingrid notices this while Astrid visits her in prison.

She can't stand the thought of Claire and her daughter being so close. So she sets out purposefully to undermine the naive, innocent Claire, playing on her self-doubts and sending her into a downward spiral.

As Astrid warns her mother to leave Claire alone, Ingrid smirks and says, "But it's such fun. Easy, but fun. In my present situation, I have to get fun where I can."

Ignoring the fact that Astrid, perhaps for the first time in her life, is in a stable loving home, Ingrid adds, "I would rather see you in the worst kind of foster hell than living with *that* woman."

Ingrid continues to prey on Claire to the point that, eventually, the depressed woman goes over the edge and commits suicide, sending Astrid to yet another foster home. Ingrid doesn't care about the fact that her daughter is happy with a woman who legitimately cares for her as a normal mother would.

She doesn't care, as a normal mother would, that her daughter will now have to suffer and go back into the foster system.

She doesn't care, as a normal person would, that Claire is a kind, decent woman who has only ever been kind to Ingrid. She simply wants to obliterate her because she's jealous.

That's the mind of an emotional predator.

An emotional predator may stir up trouble just for the fun of watching people squirm. An emotional predator may use guilt, blame, and fear on you, just to see how you'll react. An emotional predator knows how to push all of your buttons.

And an emotional predator may even choose to play the victim so that you'll never hold her accountable for her actions.

In her book *The Sociopath Next Door*, Martha Stout tells a chilling story about asking a formally diagnosed psychopath about what he wanted more than anything else in life. His answer astonished her:

> *"Oh that's easy. What I like better than anything else is when people feel sorry for me. The thing I really want more than anything else out of life is people's pity."*

This is not what you'd expect from a psychopath, but as Stout herself later explains,

> *"... the explanation is that good people will let pathetic individuals get by with murder, so to speak, and therefore any sociopath wishing to continue with his game, whatever it happens to be, should play repeatedly for none other than pity."*

Pity is a commodity for an emotional predator.

I once knew a woman who constantly played the victim in her life—to anyone who would listen. She would rip people apart behind their backs without a shred of guilt. But if you confronted her, she'd either burst into tears and deny she ever said anything, or she would run away, pretending she just couldn't take the stress of your cruel accusations.

It was a very convenient way to avoid taking any responsibility for the messes she created. She even acted like a child, using a high-pitched voice and acting helpless, as if she couldn't be trusted to tie her own shoes.

Most people's reactions to her were similar, "Oh, that poor thing, she's had such a hard life. She doesn't even know what she's doing."

But if you watched her carefully, you would see her planting gossip behind people's backs. You would catch her planting doubt and playing people—even her own kids—off against one another.

She reveled in the drama. She loved creating a crisis and the excitement that went along with it. She didn't care that people were hurt or that lives were destroyed; she just wanted the excitement of a crisis.

She was one of the worst emotional predators I've ever witnessed, and sadly enough, because she knew how to play the pity card, most people didn't have a clue that she was the one pulling the strings the whole time.

Not all emotional predators play the pity game. There are other ways they try to manipulate you, based on your weaknesses and their style.

However, the pity game is a great example of an emotional ploy that a predator can use— to get what they want from you— that a normal person would not.

Emotional predators can actually sometimes be worse than physical predators because they scheme against you covertly. They use emotional weapons while assuming the appearance of an angel in your life.

And with an emotional predator, it can often be harder (but not impossible) to see the attack coming until damage has already been done. Let's talk about how this happened to Jenna.

Jenna's Experience:

Jenna had been working at the bank for seven years. She'd started out as a personal advisor, selling mortgages, bank accounts, credit cards, and the occasional mutual fund to her customers. What she really wanted, though, was to move up to the high-end investment management side of the bank. That was what really fired her up—it was her dream job.

She'd worked hard for the last seven years to prove she could handle it. She'd taken all the required investment-licensing courses. She'd served her clients with excellence. She even made her sales quotas every week without fail.

She was so good she was assigned to train the new girl, Kelly—perhaps as her possible replacement?

Everything was falling into place. It was so close Jenna could almost taste it.

Even her boss, the branch manager, Mr. Jenkins—although he wasn't always tuned into what was going on—hinted that a big promotion was coming her way. So Jenna kept working hard, making her sales quotas and training the new girl.

Kelly was a young, slim brunette with an upturned nose, a sprinkle of freckles, and eager brown eyes. She was a bit intense but very eager to learn. She hung on Jenna's every word, making Jenna feel like a rock star. She wanted to know everything and to do it (eventually) just as well as Jenna.

During their breaks, Kelly even wanted to know about Jenna's personal life and family. Jenna found this flattering as few people working at the branch ever asked her about her life outside the bank. The two women took to spending all their break times together. Kelly was hilarious, entertaining Jenna with observations about the people they worked with.

She could imitate all their individual quirks to perfection, from Mr. Jenkins's bumbling mannerisms to Mrs. Harper's beady-eyed, condescending "Humpf!" It could sometimes border on being catty. But Kelly was young, Jenna thought, and young girls sometimes didn't know enough to be kind.

When Kelly discovered that Jenna was an avid rollerblader, she squealed, "I LOVE rollerblading, but since I'm new in town, I don't know any good trails. You have to show me!"

Jenna agreed and the two started rollerblading together on a regular basis.

Over the next few weeks, Jenna noticed that Kelly was starting to change. She seemed more down, a little depressed—at least in Jenna's presence. Kelly put up a good front in front of others at the bank. Jenna began to get concerned over Kelly's listlessness. So one morning she called Kelly into her office, shut the door, and asked her what was wrong.

After a few minutes, Kelly started crying uncontrollably and it all came out. Her boyfriend, whom she'd moved to this city to be with, had left her for another woman—her best friend, actually. Kelly had actually found them in bed together, she said, sobbing quietly into a wad of Kleenex. Now she had no idea what she was going to do or where she would stay. She had nowhere to go, and her boyfriend wanted her gone ASAP.

Jenna felt awful for the poor girl. She quickly told Kelly she could move in with her until she found her own place. Kelly lifted her tear-stained face.

"Really? You mean it? I don't want to put you out."

"It's no trouble. I'm sure you could use a friend right now anyway."

"Oh, thank you so much, Jenna! You're the best! I can't thank you enough."

Over the next few weeks Jenna actually found she liked having someone around, especially someone who was so interested in her life. She felt like Kelly was the sister she'd never had.

And Kelly needed her, too. She was an emotional wreck, crying almost every night over her broken relationship. Jenna listened to it all while handing her the Kleenex. Girl bonding. It was nice to be needed.

Kelly also asked for Jenna's advice on everything from dressing for the office to how to handle people at the bank. It was like a big-sister relationship, and Jenna was flattered that Kelly took her advice. She watched Kelly making the changes that she'd recommended to give her a more professional standing at the bank.

A few months later, Kelly moved out to her own place. Jenna was sad to see her go, but frankly, the intensity of Kelly's personality had grown a bit grating. She was looking forward to having her place to herself again.

It was around that time that Jenna noticed something a little strange. People at work were acting overly nice to her, stopping by her office to ask her if she was all right, dropping off home-baked cookies for her.

It was flattering but odd, since it had never happened before in the seven years she'd been at the bank. Even Mr. Jenkins stopped by her office one day and asked her if there was anything she'd like to talk about. Jenna was perplexed but said nothing; the bank rolled along as usual. Now, she just had to wait until her promotion came.

A few weeks later the kindness of her coworkers started to wane, and Jenna noticed they now seemed to be avoiding her. They wouldn't meet her eyes. They acted polite but never warmed to her conversation. Even Mr. Jenkins seemed to turn around and walk the other way when he saw her coming. What was going on, Jenna wondered. Was she imagining things or was she just in an episode of *The Twilight Zone?*

Thankfully, Kelly stopped by every day for a closed-door chat. She was her same, slightly intense self. And she was still thanking Jenna for being there for her in her time of need.

One day, however, she seemed concerned and asked Jenna, "Are you all right lately? You look a bit tired. Pale, you know, not yourself."

Jenna thought a moment and then shrugged. "No, I feel fine. Maybe I'm working a bit too hard, and the stress is a bit high. But I can handle it."

Kelly looked doubtful and worried as she opened the door. "Okay," she said, a bit loudly, "but just make sure you're taking good care of yourself."

Over the next week Kelly continued to insinuate that her friend was looking a bit haggard. Now that Jenna thought about it, she was looking a bit rough. Maybe she should take a week of her vacation and have some fun.

When she went to Mr. Jenkins, he hastily agreed. "Yes, yes. I think that's a good idea. You take care of yourself and take all the time you need."

Jenna left her client appointments and other duties in Kelly's capable hands and went home to relax. After a week of spa appointments, eating her favorite foods, and watching chick flicks in bed all day long, she felt refreshed and ready to get back to work.

But that's when she noticed the real change. People were avoiding her now more than ever. She felt like a leper.

Even Kelly seemed a bit distant. One day Jenna walked into Mr. Jenkins's office only to find him and Kelly in deep conversation. They both jumped, and Kelly looked like a kid caught with her hand in the cookie jar. A nagging instinct told Jenna they'd been talking about her.

Don't be silly, she told herself. *You're acting paranoid. Maybe the stress is starting to get to you.*

The Twilight Zone feeling continued, and Jenna grew tenser and tenser. She jumped at any little noise and even started being short with customers. By this time, even Kelly was nowhere to be found.

Then it happened.

Monday morning Jenna was called into a private meeting with Mr. Jenkins. The look on his face turned Jenna's blood cold. A sinking heart told her this was not the promotion she'd been expecting.

Mr. Jenkins told her to sit down and then folded his fingers into a steeple. He wore a tense expression and spoke as if he'd rehearsed this speech a hundred times the night before.

"Jenna, we know you've been going through a rough time lately, what with your personal problems and all. We've all tried to be understanding about that for months now. But unfortunately, it's gotten out of control."

"What?"

"You don't have to hide it, my dear. Kelly broke down and told me everything, how your boyfriend cheated on you with your best friend. We knew Kelly had to move in with you, but we didn't know the extent of the problem. I understand that you've been through an ordeal."

Jenna felt numb. Her brain was fuzzy and she couldn't put the pieces together fast enough. Mr. Jenkins then dropped the final bomb.

"We all have problems. However, when you start making the kinds of mistakes you've made over the past few weeks, mistakes that have cost the bank a lot of money—well, that's just not acceptable."

"Mistakes?" Jenna repeated in a fog. "What mistakes?"

"Credit lines being given to people that didn't qualify. Mortgages that were entered incorrectly into the system—you know our mortgage department had to work overtime to sort the mess out. You even gave a second mortgage to a man without his wife's knowledge—that's a huge no-no, Jenna. We might even face some legal action when she finds out her house now has a second mortgage on it. These kinds of errors are inexcusable."

Mr. Jenkins sighed and leaned back in his chair.

"I hate to do this, Jenna, but I'm going to have to let you go. I hope you can sort out your problems and get back on your feet, honestly I do. But you won't be doing it at this bank. Security is waiting outside to help you clean out your desk."

Jenna rose from the chair in a haze and walked out of Mr. Jenkins's office for the last time, all her dreams—the last seven years—down the drain.

How? How had this happened? What had happened?

The last thing she saw as she passed through the bank lobby was Kelly's face and the slight smirk she wore as she watched Jenna walk out the doors.

A couple of years later, Jenna heard through an old friend that worked at a sister bank branch that Kelly had gotten the job in investment management—the job Jenna had worked towards for over seven years.

An Emotional Predator in Action

Kelly is a great example of an emotional predator, somebody who won't harm you physically but doesn't think twice about targeting you and taking what you've worked for.

She zeroed in on Jenna from day one. Jenna had everything Kelly wanted—the job, the respect, the experience. After watching Jenna for a few weeks, she had put together a profile of Jenna's strengths and weaknesses. (This is an example of the extended interview.)

Kelly then formulated a well-laid-out plan of how to nibble away at Jenna's reputation, to start to make her look bad, and eventually, to slowly set herself up as the ultimate solution to the problem of Jenna's so-called demise—a demise that Kelly herself planned out very carefully.

She knew Jenna didn't open up much to her coworkers, so she slowly spread rumors of Jenna's boyfriend troubles. That explained why Kelly had to stay at Jenna's place. She also planted doubt in Jenna's mind, telling her she didn't look so good and suggesting a break.

She held closed-door sessions in Jenna's office to make it look like she was counseling her coworker.

When Jenna took some time off, Kelly went to work, backdating paperwork and making the 'mistakes' that Jenna supposedly had made. When Jenna came back, she didn't look over her paperwork a second time because she assumed Kelly had handled it properly. She just sent it off to be processed.

Kelly then went to Mr. Jenkins a few weeks later with her concerns and the 'proof' of Jenna's mistakes. Because she had laid the groundwork for weeks, planting doubts in people's minds, they easily drew their own conclusions that Jenna was unstable.

And to this day, Jenna is still unsure exactly what went wrong. She knows that Kelly was behind it, but she isn't sure how she could have stopped it.

What could Jenna have done? How could she have spotted this emotional predator?

By now, you can probably pick up the red flags yourself. These red flags could have warned Jenna had she known what to look for.

First of all, there was Kelly's intensity. She came on too strong and seemed to have an almost 'single white female' obsession with Jenna's life.

While Jenna found this flattering at first, her instincts were still warning her that something did not fit. (Recall the fourth area of awareness—incongruency—looking for what doesn't fit?)

Secondly, Kelly wanted to move in with her after only a few months of knowing each other. She used the boyfriend sob story—the pity play.

But if Jenna had been paying attention, she would have realized that Kelly was new in town. How could she have a boyfriend AND a best friend already? Again, this was something else that didn't add up. Her story didn't add up and the details did not agree.

Jenna had also ignored the fact that her coworkers were acting differently around her.

She was too focused on doing her job to stop and ask a simple question of her boss or her coworkers. By saying nothing, she was unknowingly confirming their impression of her problems.

She also ignored her instincts, feeling more and more tense, but not sure why. She could feel other people's hostility towards her, but she still said nothing. Again, this just fed into their growing resentment and belief that she was making major mistakes.

Finally, when it all went down, Jenna was blindsided by the accusations. By that point it was too late, and seven years of hard work were down the drain. There was nothing she could have done.

You may have run into someone like Kelly before—a predator who looks like a nice person on the outside, but once they're done with you, you're just as blindsided as Jenna was.

We're going to talk about how you can spot these kinds of people in the next chapter on sociopaths and narcissists. We'll go a little further into exploring the mind of a predator, whether physical or emotional. With a little knowledge and skill, you'll be able to identify them and steer clear of being their next victim.

Important Points:

- ◊ Predators don't think like you.
- ◊ If someone has crossed the line of polite society by targeting you, they will not adhere to the rules of polite society once they have you.
- ◊ Don't expect mercy, honesty, or honor if a predator comes after you.
- ◊ About 5 percent of the population could be classified as an 'emotionally disturbed person' at any one time. By these odds alone, chances are high that you'll run into a few predators in your lifetime.
- ◊ If you are targeted by a predator, be prepared to fight like hell until they are unable to come after you and you can get away.

◊ There are predators that are more subtle. They attack you psychologically and emotionally, but not physically.

◊ You can often spot emotional predators by using your awareness skills (what doesn't fit), looking for the pity play, and listening to your instincts when things feel off about a person.

Chapter 8 –
The Slow Poisoning of Sociopaths and Narcissists in Your Life

By Kate O'Neill

"... sociopaths are noted especially for their shallowness of emotion, the hollow and transient nature of any affectionate feelings they may claim to have, a certain breathtaking callousness. They have no trace of empathy and no genuine interest in bonding emotionally with a mate."
— Martha Stout, The Sociopath Next Door

"The sadistic narcissist perceives himself as Godlike, ruthless and devoid of scruples, capricious and unfathomable, emotion-less and non-sexual, omniscient, omnipotent and omni-present, a plague, a devastation, an inescapable verdict." — Sam Vaknin, Self-Proclaimed Narcissist

In the last chapter we talked about predators that brutally attack you or come after you, usually with the intent to physically harm you.

But how do you spot a predator who wants to destroy your life from the inside out? How do you avoid becoming a victim of an emotional predator, a sociopath, or a narcissist?

In this chapter we're going to expose two very common types of predators: sociopaths (also called psychopaths) and narcissists.

We're going to talk about how you can identify these people and see them coming so that you can get away and avoid becoming their next victim.

Note: In this book we use the terms 'sociopath' and 'psychopath' interchangeably. According to some experts there are differences between the two. Other experts think they are essentially the same.

However, for the purposes of this book, the slight differences between the two are not as important as how to identify them in the first place. So the two terms will be used interchangeably here.

What Exactly is a Sociopath?

We usually think of sociopaths as criminally insane monsters like Charles Manson or Ted Bundy—and they can certainly take that form. Many criminals are sociopaths; however, not all sociopaths are criminals.

There are also what you might call 'lesser' sociopaths walking around that may be content to con you, steal from you, or torture you with mind games just for the fun of it.

They could be people like Kelly in the previous chapter, bent on destroying your reputation and stealing everything you've worked for.

They could be that person the next table over in Starbucks who walks off with your laptop when you get up to order a second latte. They could be a con artist that you met on an internet-dating site who plans to charm you and then steal your identity.

The main point is that a sociopath has no conscience. (Recall from the last chapter—they don't think like you.)

"These often charming—but always deadly—individuals have a clinical name: psychopaths. Their hallmark is a <u>stunning lack of conscience</u>; their game is self-gratification at the other person's expense. Many spend time in prison, but many do not. All take far more than they give." — Robert D. Hare, PhD, Without Conscience: The Disturbing World of Psychopaths Among Us

Sociopaths often see themselves as above the law. They see you as a pawn in their own personal game, and they will think nothing of using you to get what they want.

How do you protect yourself from a sociopath? The best way is to be able to identify one before you get too involved with him or her and get as far away from them as you can.

With that in mind, here are the top 11 signs of a sociopath or psychopath:

Top 11 Signs of a Sociopath

#1: They're Charming and Magnetic: These people can be charming and charismatic, especially at first. They may be physically attractive and they know how to use it.

They use their magnetic personality to draw people into their circle. Hitler, for example, had an almost demonically powerful charisma when he spoke that could charm thousands of people at once. Many cult leaders also often display this heightened charisma.

#2: They Are Intense and Spontaneous: Many people like to spice things up and do crazy, spur-of-the-moment things. But sociopaths have an intense, insatiable hunger for excitement almost ALL the time.

They absolutely cannot stand boredom or monotony. This leads them to do crazy things. They may even encourage you to do crazy things with them as well.

They may experiment with drugs, jump from job to job, or take on a job that gives them a constant adrenaline buzz. They may commit crimes just for the fun of seeing if they can get away with it. They may mentally torture people just to watch their reaction.

#3: They are Grandiose and Ego-Centric: Sociopaths truly believe the world revolves around them. They often display a heightened sense of their own importance in the world, as in: "I'm the reincarnation of Jesus" or "I am the One chosen to bring about the coming of a Divine New Order."

Because of this, they feel self-entitled to do whatever they want, including use people as pawns and then throw them away.

They truly feel they have special skills beyond what the normal population has. As such, they should not be held down by silly things like the obligation to pay debts or act according to the rules of polite society. The rules should not apply to them because they are special.

#4: They Feel No Shame, Guilt, or Remorse: This goes back to having no conscience as we discussed above. They don't feel the consequent shame for their actions that a normal person would. If you catch them in a lie, they will show no remorse; they'll simply ignore you and keep spinning their tales in a new direction.

Having no conscience allows them to turn on people on a dime and betray them at a second's notice. This includes people who have been with them for years.

Once they have no use for you, you are dispensable. The question they face is how to get rid of you in the cleanest, most trouble-free way possible.

#5: They Lie Constantly and Outrageously: Sociopaths lie constantly, sometimes for protection but many times just for fun.

Have you ever met someone whose stories seemed more outrageous than anyone else's?

Instead of getting mugged, they got pulled into a satanic cult ritual? Instead of going on a cruise, they had a millionaire friend who chartered them a yacht?

Instead of having a rebellious teenager, their kid was now a drug dealer being targeted by local gangs? Instead of trying to write a book, they had a major publisher sending them advances, begging them to finish the great American novel?

These may all be true stories, but when you see an ongoing pattern of too-dramatic-to-be-true stories, it's a warning sign. And as stated above, if you catch them in a lie, they usually won't admit it or show any remorse for it.

#6: They Have to Win at All Costs: These people have to be right—about everything. Even when caught in their own lies, they will attack you for daring to expose them. Their main objective is to win, no matter the cost to others.

#7: They Tend to Be Highly Intelligent: This isn't a given. However, many well-known sociopaths are highly intelligent. With this intelligence comes a haughty arrogance, which feeds into their belief that they have every right to use people for their own ends.

#8: They are Incapable of Love or Empathy: Because they have no conscience, they literally cannot empathize with others' feelings. Consequently, they are incapable of loving anyone. They may know how to put on an 'act' of loving, but when you separate their words from their actions, they don't add up.

#8: They Never Apologize: Because they're always right, they never apologize. Even if they are shown to be in the wrong, you'll never hear them say, "I'm sorry."

"I have no desire whatever to reform myself. My only desire is to reform people who try to reform me, and I believe the only way to reform people is to kill 'em. My motto is 'Rob 'em'all, rape 'em all and kill 'em all." — Carl Panzram, serial killer and sociopath

#9: They Take *No* Responsibility for Their Actions (Unless It Makes Them Look Good): In fact, they will usually frame all of their problems—or crimes—as somebody else's fault:

"You made me hit you with all your crying."

"If you weren't so fat, I wouldn't have to cheat on you."

"Men like you deserve to be conned because all you want is sex."

#10: They Have a Very Loose Grip on Reality: Because they have no conscience, you may hear them make a statement and think, "What? Are they for real? How can anybody say that?"

What sounds ludicrous to you may seem perfectly normal to them. For example, they may say something like (à la Charles Manson) they can kill people with their minds.

They may threaten (as one sociopath did to Chuck years ago) to send their 'armies of darkness' after you.

Another example of this is seen in a comment from German serial killer, Rudoph Pleil:

"Every man has his passion; some like whist, I prefer killing people."

This would almost be funny because it's so insanely ludicrous. It's something right out of a Hannibal Lector movie. You know that nobody in his right mind thinks this way. But a sociopath with no concept of reality might think it's perfectly normal.

#11: They Will Turn on You if Questioned or Challenged: Many sociopaths will display intense, almost over-the-top anger when questioned. They may attack your character out of the blue or turn on you for daring to challenge them.

Chuck once heard from a fellow martial artist about a fairly popular instructor. This particular instructor was teaching at a seminar years ago when a student asked him a simple question about the effectiveness of a technique he was demonstrating.

This instructor, in a sudden and intense fit of rage at being questioned, turned on the student and screamed, "You DARE to question the Master?" He humiliated the student (who, by the way, had paid several hundred dollars to be there) all because this man asked a simple question.

So those are 11 warning signs or red flags to look for to spot a sociopath.

While not all sociopaths will display these 11 red flags, they will display many of them. By keeping your eyes open for these signs, you can begin to spot sociopaths, or those with sociopathic tendencies, as they come your way.

George Simon has a great description of these types of predators in his book *In Sheep's Clothing:*

> *These characters are radically different from most people. Their lack of conscience is unnerving. They tend to see themselves as superior creatures for whom the inferior, common man is rightful prey. They are the **most extreme manipulators** or con artists who thrive on exploiting and abusing others. They can be charming and disarming. As highly skilled predators, they study the vulnerabilities of their prey carefully and are capable of the most heinous acts of victimization with no sense of remorse or regret.*

How Do You Deal with a Sociopath?

If you suspect someone of having sociopathic tendencies, there are a few things you can do.

First of all, check their facts. If they tell you outrageous stories, check them out. See if they are indeed telling the truth. Watch them and see if their actions line up with their words.

Watch for the patterns in behavior like constant, grandiose stories or risk-taking behaviors.

Question them. Do they get offended? Do they turn and attack you for questioning them? Do they lie and show no remorse when called on it? This is not a good sign, especially if this person is a leader of any type of group.

Now, one or two red flags do not equal a sociopath; it could just mean that person is an ego-maniac, arrogant, cruel, or overly selfish. They may even just be having a really bad day and are acting childish.

The key is to watch them and look for numerous red flags popping up—*look for clusters*. If this person is truly dangerous, you will see a steady cluster of red flags on a regular basis. If you start to see this, the best way to protect yourself is to remove yourself from the situation. Get away from them if you can. Start putting up and enforcing boundaries if you can't get away. (We'll talk more about this in a later chapter.)

And one thing you should never do?

Don't ever expect that person to change.

Don't expect to reform them. Don't hope that they will suddenly start to empathize with you or 'see the light' and change their ways. They won't.

And it's not worth it for you to waste your time trying. Chances are that you'll get hurt in the process.

Narcissists: Emotional Predators with a Conscience

A related category of people that are perhaps not as dangerous—although they can certainly be just as harmful—as sociopaths are narcissists.

We usually think of a narcissist as someone who just loves themselves a little too much, or maybe someone who is annoyingly egotistical.

However, most experts feel that narcissism is a spectrum disorder—we all have some healthy levels of narcissism, or self-love, which is normal.

But there are others on the opposite end of that spectrum, those that can be termed as personality disordered, or NPD (narcissistic personality disorder). And these people can be downright devastating.

The term *narcissism* itself comes from the Greek myth about a handsome young man named Narcissus. He was loved and admired by many, but loved no one but himself.

He rejected the love of a wood nymph named Echo and instead fell in love with his own reflection in a pool of water. He was so in love with his reflection that he refused to move or leave it. He eventually withered and died, leaving a flower in his place.

NPD is a term used to describe an individual who is excessively preoccupied with self, so much so that they often misuse and harm others in order to maintain this image of themselves.

According to the Mayo Clinic website:

> *"Narcissistic personality disorder is a mental disorder in which people have an inflated sense of their own importance and a deep need for admiration. Those with narcissistic personality disorder believe that they're superior to others and have little regard for other people's feelings. But behind this mask of ultra-confidence lies a fragile self-esteem, vulnerable to the slightest criticism."*

(http://www.mayoclinic.com/health/narcissistic-personality-disorder/DS00652)

Unlike sociopaths who have no conscience, narcissists do understand when they've done something wrong (which is seen in their frequent attempts to cover up their harmful actions). However, that doesn't stop them from doing it.

The main defining feature of someone with NPD is a complete lack of empathy for other human beings, including their children and spouses. Everyone in a narcissist's life is sacrificed to maintain their fragile image of themselves.

Symptoms of this disorder, as defined by the DSM-IV-TR (*Diagnostic and Statistical Manual of Mental Disorders*) include:

◊ Reacting to criticism with anger, humiliation, or shaming of others

◊ Taking advantage of others to reach their own goals

◊ Exaggerating their own importance, achievements, and talents

◊ Imagining unrealistic fantasies of success, beauty, power, intelligence, or romance

◊ Needing constant attention and positive reinforcement from others (also known as 'narcissistic supply')

◊ Becoming jealous of others easily—including their own children and spouses

◊ Lacking empathy and disregarding the feelings of others

◊ Being obsessed with self

◊ Pursuing mainly selfish goals

◊ Have trouble keeping healthy relationships

◊ Becoming easily hurt and rejected

◊ Setting unrealistic goals

◊ Wanting 'the best' of everything

◊ Appearing unemotional

Experts believe that narcissists maintain an image—or a mask—to hide a brittle, fragile self-esteem. They create a 'false self' so to speak, and everyone around them becomes the 'mirror' which is supposed to reflect back this false image they want to see.

For example, a parent with NPD may see their children as extensions of themselves, existing solely and exclusively to serve the parent. They may expect the child to take care of them emotionally and physically, constantly sacrificing their own needs to serve the parent's needs. Children raised by these kinds of parents inevitably suffer immense physical and emotional damage.

If you have a friend with NPD, they may talk incessantly about themselves, expect you to admire them endlessly, go where they want to go, and be available whenever they want you. They never give back, and if someone else gossips about you, they'll be the first to throw you under the bus.

There are different types of narcissists; many of them seek power, fame, and prestige in public arenas. However, others may seek admiration from more local sources, like their children or from their job.

So you may find a narcissist in a job as a school teacher, a psychologist, or a pastor—any job that gives them a sense of superiority over others. (That's not saying that all teachers, psychologists, or pastors are narcissists; these are just examples of jobs that tend to attract people with NPD.)

If you live with somebody with NPD, it gets even worse. According to an article at www.medicalnewstoday.com:

> *"Family members of somebody with NPD describe the sufferer as controlling, egotistical and forever dissatisfied with what anybody around them does. No matter what happens, the narcissist will blame others and make them*

feel guilty for all their problems.

They are described as having short fuses, losing their tempers at the slightest provocation, or turning their backs and giving people the 'silent treatment.' Some can be physically and sexually abusive."

(Read the whole article at http://www.medicalnewstoday.com/articles/9741.php)

While someone with NPD may not be an axe murderer or even as dangerously manipulative as a sociopath, they can definitely do a lot of damage once you've let them into your life.

Plus, because they will never admit that they have a problem, it's very hard for a narcissist to get diagnosed. Most people with NPD are diagnosed from afar—when the victim of the narcissist goes to a psychologist to try and recover from what was done to them by the narcissist.

Many victims of narcissists suffer silently and never even know it because the narcissist is so great at blaming their victims for their mistakes that the victims believe it's all their fault.

If you're unsure if you're dealing with a narcissist or not (or even with someone that may have narcissistic tendencies), here are seven signs to watch out for.

Top Seven Signs You're Dealing with a Narcissist:

#1: They Show No Interest in Your Life: It's always a red flag when I meet someone in a social setting for the first time and they don't ask one question about me, even though I may ask them several dozen about themselves. Someone with NPD doesn't care about your life, so they generally won't show interest in it.

The only exception here is when they think they can get something out of you or that you can help them in some way. In that case, they will ask you questions to find out what you can offer them (e.g., your experience, contacts, start-up capital, etc.).

#2: They Are Right about Everything: Ever meet someone who knows everything about everything? Even if they worked at McDonald's and ran into Tiger Woods, they'd be instructing him on how to change his golf swing and do it the 'right' way for his next game.

I was once invited to a cottage by a friend of a friend. My host for the weekend—whom I'd met only once before—turned out to have very strong narcissistic tendencies.

It had taken me three hours to drive up to the cottage from my home. When I arrived, this person then proceeded to inform me that I had not, in fact, driven three hours—it must have been two hours.

Why? Because he owned the cottage and therefore he knew how long the drive would be. And according to him, it should take no more than two hours.

I was astonished as this man corrected me and told me (not suggested) that I had, in fact, driven only two hours—not three as I had just stated. I should also mention that he never knew—or cared to ask—where I lived or what traffic had been like on the drive up. Narcissists are always right.

#3: They Act Superior to Everyone: Narcissists know better than everyone. They are better than everyone. They are constantly waiting and looking for other people to screw up or make mistakes so that they can talk about them behind their backs and feel superior.

A good friend of mine was raised with a narcissistic mother and sister. She said to me one day:

"You know, family get-togethers are not fun at my house. My mom and sister are just waiting to pounce on anything I say so they can make fun of me and feel better about themselves. They're like scorpions, just waiting to sting.

And heaven forbid if I bring my boyfriend over. He's not as educated as my sister, so my sister will set him up, lay out the trap with a comment or two. And when my boyfriend takes the bait, my mom and sister both get these smirks on their faces.

I know the moment my boyfriend leaves my Mom will be crowing about how stupid he is."

#4 They Gaslight: Every narcissist gaslights—and it's one of the most insidious forms of emotional abuse you can experience. This is basically when the narcissist lies to you in order to make you question and doubt your own experience of reality.

The term 'gaslight' actually came from a movie made in 1944 of the same name starring Ingrid Bergman and Charles Boyer. In it, the scheming husband tries to drive his wife mad by secretly, slowly turning the gaslights down and then telling her that she's imagining it.

If you've ever confronted someone about something they've done to you only to have them say, "I never did that!" or "You're imagining things!" you've been gaslighted.

If you've ever heard the phrase, "It never happened like that" (when you know it did), you've been gaslighted.

If you've ever been told, "I don't remember that. Are you sure you aren't making that up?" (when you know you're not), you've been gaslighted.

Both sociopaths and narcissists gaslight constantly.

That's not to say if somebody does this, they're automatically a narcissist or a sociopath. Sometimes people really do forget what they said or did. But again, look for repeating clusters of behavior.

A friend of mine, Sarah, gave me a great example of the gaslighting done to her by her mother over the course of about 10 years.

Sarah always suspected that her older sister Erica didn't like her. She wasn't sure why; she just got that feeling whenever they were together.

Erica never reached out to her, never called her, never invited her over to her home (which was 10 minutes away). At their parent's house, Erica constantly gave subtle digs to her sister, criticizing everything from Sarah's cooking skills and fashion choices to the new diet she was trying.

Sarah's mom heard it all but said nothing. Sarah's mom was, in fact, a narcissist who would have done anything to maintain the perfect family image she'd built up over the years: She still expected Sarah to invite Erica to her home, to include her in every family event, and to even throw her a birthday party—despite the fact that Erica had never even sent Sarah so much as a card for her birthday.

Sarah would periodically get fed up with her older sister's behavior. Erica's actions were a blaring horn, telling Sarah that her sister didn't like her; she was even malevolent towards Sarah. But whenever Sarah would bring it up to her mother, her mother would always tell Sarah that she was imagining things.

She might then go on to tell Sarah a story of how Erica was bragging about how wonderful her sister was just the other week. A week later, Sarah's mother might relate something Erica had supposedly said about how glad she was to have a sister like Sarah.

Sarah was being gaslighted.

Watching her sister's actions told her that Erica was hostile towards her. But her mother—in the interests of keeping the perfect family image together—was lying and telling Sarah things to make her question her own experiences with her sister.

Sarah endured her sister's hateful digs for over 10 years until it got so bad that Sarah finally had to trust her own perception and walk away from her acidic, jealous sister. Not only that, but she was badly hurt when she realized how masterfully her own mother had gaslighted her—all for the sake of keeping the perfect family image intact.

#5: They Project Their Faults onto You: When people project, they assign to you characteristics they themselves have but aren't willing to admit. So an arrogant, judgmental, narcissistic friend might accuse you of getting up on your 'high horse' and looking down your nose at everybody.

A serial cheater may accuse you of stepping out on him. A woman with weight issues may accuse her normal-weight daughter of having an eating disorder.

That's projection. Because a narcissist will never take responsibility for themselves or admit to making a mistake, they will project these mistakes onto you. Don't fall for it.

"Since they must deny their own badness, they must perceive others as bad. They project their own evil onto the world. The evil attack others instead of facing their own failures." — M Scott Peck, *People of the Lie*

#6: They Invade Your Boundaries: This can be physically, as in helping themselves to your food, your home, or your money. It can also be emotionally.

They may act entitled to your attention and time. They may act as if your main reason for living is to fulfill their wants and needs alone. They may be offended, for example, if they call you on a

Friday night and you're busy—as in "How DARE you have a life outside of me?"

#7: They Play the Victim—Constantly: One amazingly effective tactic of the narcissist is to play the victim. It's a popular ploy because most people fall for it. After all, who doesn't want to help someone who is down on their luck?

And 'pathetic' people can get away with so much more than normal people. We think, "They're going through such a hard time, I should cut them some slack" or "I'm sure she's only acting that way because she was abused."

They may give you the sob story to end all sob stories. Their boyfriend cheated. Their dog died. Their last three bosses were mean to them. Their kids never visit them. Their best friend stole from them.

That's not to say we shouldn't help people who are down on their luck. Everybody needs some help when going through a rough patch in life. The key here is the 'constant' part. These people are always victims. Every time you talk to them it's a new sob story.

The key is that by watching them over time, you'll start to notice that they take absolutely no responsibility for their lives. They want to complain and milk you for your sympathy, but when it comes to lifting a finger to get out of their self-dug pit, they won't do it.

Instead, they'll shift blame. They'll blame everyone else, including you, for their hard times: You didn't help them enough. You weren't a good enough friend. You didn't anticipate what they needed. You didn't fix it all for them. You didn't share your wealth.

Be very careful of these kinds of people. They will suck you dry of everything they can get, whether it's your sympathy, your money, your time, or your physical aid.

How Can You Protect Yourself against a Narcissist?

In a word, *run*. Get away from them if possible. Cut off contact and don't go back.

Don't try to engage them. Don't try to make them feel sorry for hurting you. Don't try to change them. And don't bother confronting them—all you'll do is give them something to use against you in the future.

If you can't get away from them, you're going to have to be very good at building and enforcing your own personal boundaries. For example, you may decide to lay down a time boundary and see them for only an hour at a time once a week.

You may decide you will see these people only on holidays and birthdays. You may decide to see them in public places but never allow them into your home.

The most important thing with a narcissist is to realize how damaging they can be. Unlike a physical attacker, a prolonged relationship with a narcissist is like a slow poisoning of your life—continue at your own risk.

Important Points:

- ◊ Predators don't always attack physically; there are far more predators who will try to hurt you emotionally and psychologically.

- ◊ Sociopaths are people who have no conscience. They will not think twice about using you for their own ends.

- ◊ Sociopaths have very definite characteristics you can spot, such as heightened charm, pathological lying, over-the-top dramatic stories, having a loose grip on reality, and never taking responsibility for their actions.

◊ Narcissists are similar to sociopaths with the exception that they do have a conscience—they just ignore it much of the time.

◊ Narcissists are characterized by the inability to feel empathy for other people, including their own families.

◊ Narcissists will hurt you in subtle ways like gaslighting, projecting, playing the victim, and disrespecting your boundaries.

◊ If you suspect someone of having sociopathic or narcissistic tendencies, don't try to change them. Your best bet is to get away or at least lay down very firm boundaries.

Chapter 9 –
Body Language – What Are *You* Saying to the People around You?

By Chuck O'Neill

"60 percent of all human communication is nonverbal body language. 30 percent is your tone, so that means 90 percent of what you're saying ain't coming out of your mouth." — Will Smith in Hitch

"What you do speaks so loud that I cannot hear what you say."
— *Ralph Waldo Emerson*

What kind of message are you sending to other people? To your friends? To your kids? To coworkers? To predators? You're actually saying a lot more than you think, without even saying a word.

The next skill in our psychological self-defense arsenal is the first of the B's in the ABCs—Body Language. By learning how to use body language to send the right message, you can save yourself from becoming a victim in many cases.

That's what this chapter is about—how to use your own body language to send the right message and avert attacks. In the next chapter we'll cover the second aspect of body language—how to read other people's body language to identify dangerous situations and people.

So What Is Body Language – and Is It Really That Important?

Body language is much more important than most people realize. Whether you know it or not, you're always communicating to the people around you. And you're always observing—even if subconsciously—the body language of others around you.

Body language can be anything from the placement of your hands on a table, to the angle of your feet while in conversation, to the brief scratching your nose as you explain your point of view, to the crossing of your legs when you're out on a blind date.

According to former FBI agent and body language expert Joe Navarro, as much as 80 percent of our interaction with others is through nonverbal communication, or body language. Some experts claim that up to 93 percent of all communication is nonverbal.

When we talk about body language, we're not just talking about movement of your body parts; we're also talking about nonverbal communication.

Although some experts like to separate the two, for practical purposes in this book I'll be including other nonverbal communication signals under this 'B' skill of body language.

Nonverbal communication can be things like:

◊ tone of voice

◊ volume of voice

◊ facial expressions

◊ personal space or proximity to another person

◊ eye movement and intensity of gaze

◊ outward appearance and clothing choices

◊ sudden changes in physical or emotional energy

◊ the agreement between someone's words and facial expression or body movement

The Benefits of Reading Body Language

Body language and nonverbal communication can be used in practically every situation you face, not only to warn you against danger. It can be used from the boardroom to the bedroom, and everything in between.

For example, whenever I do a seminar, I'm always reading body language.

When people are leaning forward, nodding, and laughing at my jokes, I know they're interested in what I'm saying. I know I'm on the right path.

However, if they're leaning back, looking around the room, or picking imaginary lint off their pants, I know that their interest is waning. That's a cue to move on to other topics that they would be more interested in or to engage them in another way.

Kate, when she was single, used body language to read her dates all the time. In fact, she told me years after we were married that she knew I was interested in her the first night we met (and I thought I'd been playing it cool!).

How? She read my body language.

The night we met, Kate had been having coffee with a girlfriend at a local coffee shop. Her girlfriend, it turned out, had met me through a mutual friend years ago. So on seeing me, she invited me to join them, much to Kate's dismay.

Kate had no interest in sitting down with some strange guy. She just wanted to enjoy her coffee and chocolate cake. Consequently, she had not been impressed by my intrusion into her girl-bonding, coffee-talk time—a fact made very obvious to me when she said very little and let her friend take over the conversation.

Her friend and I spent a couple of hours recalling old times, flirting and laughing it up. I kept trying to bring Kate into the conversation, but I knew she wasn't having any of it.

Then it happened; I gave my interest away without even realizing it.

She was sitting to my right and her girlfriend was seated across the table from me. As I continued talking to her friend, I casually turned my right foot towards Kate and rested it on the bottom rung of her chair.

That was it.

That's the moment she knew I was interested. My body language had given me away. The rest, as they say, is history.

You can use body language in lots of different situations, not just for self-protection. You can also use it to improve your relationships, achieve goals, make more sales, find great friendships, and get more of what you want overall. You can use it to:

◊ negotiate a business contract in your favor

◊ find the right new employee for your company

◊ discern if a person is interested in you romantically or just as a friend

◊ send the message to a potential predator that you're not a good victim ('fail' the interview)

◊ get someone to invest with you

◊ pass a job interview with flying colors

◊ discern whether a potential mate is sincere or a serial cheater

◊ find the right babysitter for your kids

◊ convince new clients to choose your services over your competition

◊ separate out serious predators from the simply obnoxious

You can even use it to understand your sullen, mouth-shut-tighter-than-a-drum teenager. (Okay, there are some limits here.)

Understanding body language can open up incredible new doors for you. And because the vast majority of people don't actually know how to read it, developing this skill can also give you the edge wherever you go.

The field of body language is huge, much too broad for a few chapters in this book. So I'd encourage you to undertake your own study of this subject. Kate runs a blog called **BodyLanguageMatters.com** that you can also visit to learn more.

In the next couple of chapters you'll find a basic primer about body language, especially as it relates to psychological self-defense.

So let's start with some key guidelines for reading body language and nonverbal communication.

Key Guidelines for Reading Body Language:

#1: Read Body Language in Clusters: You can't draw a specific conclusion from one or two signs. You have to look at multiple signs that all agree with each other (and even then you can only start to form a hypothesis).

For example, you may be in a business negotiation and the person across from you crosses their arms. This is a universal body language signal that says this person is hostile, in disagreement with what you're saying, or closed to your proposal.

However, they might also be cold.

They may be wearing a shirt that's too tight and feeling self-conscious about it. They may just feel more comfortable in that position.

You can't conclude that just because they cross their arms your negotiations are going badly.

However, if you also notice that they lean back away from you, stop meeting your gaze, and shake their head back and forth at your comments, that's a cluster that says they may indeed be turning hostile.

Here's another example from the dating world.

Let's say you're on a date and the woman of your dreams just crossed her legs away from you (which can be a sign of disinterest). This doesn't automatically mean that you just said something to turn her off.

It could mean, for example, that she's had her legs crossed towards you for twenty minutes and they're now hurting her in that position. She's crossing her legs away because it's physically more comfortable for her.

But if you notice her leaning back in her chair, glancing covertly at her watch, giving you a bland smile that doesn't quite reach her eyes, that's a good cluster of body language signals that tells you she isn't interested.

So you have to read body language in clusters. When several signs are in agreement, you can start to form a hypothesis. (You still can't be 100 percent sure of your conclusion because humans are so complex.) If you want to, you can then test that hypothesis for confirmation.

In the business negotiation example above, for instance, you could stop and ask the person across from you if they agree. In the date situation you could stop talking and see if they show any interest in engaging you.

#2: Consider the Context of the Situation: You also have to consider the context of the situation when reading people. For example, if it's a hot summer day and you're questioning someone in a building with no air conditioning, they may be sweating—not because they're lying—but because, in fact, they're hot.

Excess blinking is also a common sign of someone who is lying. However, if you know they have a problem with dry eyes or they've recently had laser eye surgery or they are under a lot of unusual stress (like in the witness box or on TV), you're going to want to consider that before jumping to the conclusion that they're lying.

#3: Consider the Person's Culture: The third thing to keep in mind is the person's culture. For example, there are certain European cultures where it's perfectly normal to stand very close to someone—much closer than someone in a North American culture would consider polite.

In Muslim cultures, it's considered inappropriate for people of the opposite sex to have anything more than very brief eye contact. In certain Asian cultures, long extended eye contact between men can be considered a challenge.

So it's very important to consider the person's culture when reading their body language.

So to summarize:

#1: Read Body Language in Clusters

#2: Read Body Language in Context

#3: Read Body Language Considering the Culture

What Message Are You Sending?

Have you ever stopped to ask what message you're sending to others? The good news is that you can control that message. With a few simple tweaks, you can make sure you're sending the message YOU want to relay.

So in terms of self-defense, you want to use your body language to tell a potential predator "I'm not the one you're looking for. I'll be too much trouble to attack."

How would you do this?

It depends on the situation. Let's say you're on the street, for example, walking in an unfamiliar area. You can stand up straight, walk confidently, and scan your area for threats. Don't wear anything that will limit your hearing (e.g., an iPod) or your sight (e.g., a hat that clouds your line of vision). Talk on your phone only if you need to and resist the urge to text.

If a stranger approaches you, look him straight in the eye and don't back down. He may just decide to continue on his way.

Remember, he doesn't know you.

For all he knows, you could be a black belt in karate or an off-duty police officer. He's reading your body language for signals that you are a weak and unaware victim. So by doing these things, you're saying, "I don't fit into the victim category."

Or let's say you're a social worker visiting a new client. You're going to a home you've never been to before. You'll want to consider everything—from your choice of clothing, to how far you stand from the door, to how you greet the client for the first time.

For example, if you're a woman, you may want to avoid wearing anything too overtly sexy (plunging V-neck sweaters, short skirts, high heels, etc.) and go for a conservative pantsuit that gives you a good range of motion.

(I realize this may not be a popular topic with women, and yes, I agree you should be able to wear what you want in a perfect world. However, this isn't a perfect world, and a predator will be sizing you up based on what you wear. You also want to wear clothes that give you a good range of motion and are easy to run in if you have to get away fast.)

You may also want to position yourself a safe distance away from the door when you ring the bell so that somebody will think twice about grabbing you and pulling you in. Choosing a seat in the home with your back to the wall ensures nobody can approach you from behind. Sitting close to an exit ensures you can escape quickly if necessary.

Using a firm, confident handshake when meeting the client relays you are strong and not easily intimidated.

Looking around the home (in a friendly way) when you enter makes it obvious you're aware of your environment. And projecting calm, strong energy as you meet with your client also sends a signal that you're nobody's victim.

So those are some examples of how you can use your body language to 'fail' the predator interview and send the right message. In any situation you enter, especially those where you suspect there may be trouble, I'd encourage you first to think of ways you can send a message of strength.

Remember our real estate agent, Cheryl, back in chapter six, who failed her interview? There were several ways she used her body language to turn her predator off.

First of all, she waited until the man had wandered away from her, into the dining room, before she turned her back on him to return to the kitchen. She turned and faced him squarely when he came into the kitchen where she was standing.

She used her eyes to look directly at him and send the message that she was wary and suspicious of his actions. She didn't come across looking like a very good victim.

Now contrast that with Kevin in chapter two, who got jumped and mugged while walking across his university campus. Although he didn't know it, he used his own body language to attract a predator.

He was listening to his iPod (effectively cutting off his sense of hearing, making him easy to approach). He was hunched over (making him appear weak and small).

He was looking at the ground (cutting off his sense of sight, again making him easy to approach). He was clearly not aware of his surroundings, not looking around or scanning the area. His body language worked against him and made him an easy target.

So while every situation is different, there are some common ways you can use your body language to send a message of strength and tell a predator that you're going to be more trouble than you're worth.

Here are some common ways to do this:

◊ Display obvious situational awareness by looking around and scanning the area. Don't block your senses with things like iPods, texting, or talking on phones.

◊ Walk confidently.

◊ Shake hands firmly.

◊ Take up as much physical space as possible (i.e. stand up tall, head raised, shoulders back and not slouched, feet shoulder-length apart and not crossed).

◊ Look people in the eye when meeting and talking.

◊ Dress appropriately for the situation (i.e. a sexy dress may be fine for a hot date with your boyfriend but for an office meeting with your conservative male boss, it sends the wrong message).

◊ Fit into your surroundings as much as possible without standing out when in a potentially dangerous situation.

The Benefits of Blending In

That last point is one that many people don't think about, and it can cause confusion because you're always being told to do the opposite.

We live in a world that tells you to stand out, be original, the most beautiful, the most attractive, the most winning, the most famous person in the room. Be a star and get attention. Be crazy and get noticed.

While that may be fine for people gunning for a reality-TV spot, if you're going into a potentially dangerous situation, it can get you killed. You have to consider the situation, especially if it's an unknown situation, and determine what you can do to fit in (or at least not to stand out).

For example, take Salma and Stacey from chapter two. They dressed to get men's attention in their own country, which was fine, fun, and harmless.

But they did the same thing in a foreign country without realizing how much it made them stand out (vs. the local women).

Just being a stunning blonde, white woman at a five-star resort in a poor country where 95 percent of people are tanned with dark hair will make you stand out. But when you add a 'party-girl' persona into the mix, you're painting a bull's-eye on your back.

The two girls got noticed all right, and they were kidnapped and sold into the sex trade as a result.

(Please note that I am not saying in any way that they deserved what happened. Nobody deserves to be a victim of a crime—ever. I'm just pointing out that if they had been more aware of their surroundings and taken steps to fit in as much as they could, they may not have been such a prime target for the bad guys.)

My own Jamaican episode also shows an epic failure of this principle. While I eventually did become aware of my situation, I didn't respect the fact that I was in a foreign country (with social rules and areas I wasn't familiar with).

I clearly dressed like a tourist, not a local. And I charged down into an area that was basically locals only without realizing that in this environment, my wife and I stuck out like sore thumbs.

A good friend of mine is a cop in one of the toughest parts of Toronto, Canada. He gave me another example of this principle in action.

There's a well-known, well-respected university in a rough area of town where my friend works. Most kids who go to this school are not local. They come from other countries or provinces and have no clue their campus is in the middle of a very poor area, an area rife with gangs and street violence.

My friend told me that one of the biggest problems the police had in this area was continuous muggings of these students both on and off campus.

The students who came to stay on the university campus were usually from middle- to upper-class families. They had lots of money, the best clothes, and the latest electronic gadgets.

They'd go wandering around the university campus late at night alone—or many times off the campus—and get mugged and jumped by the local gangs for whatever they had—shoes, iPods, iPhones, Blackberries, laptops, designer purses, etc.

It was a common problem, and sometimes the attacks were pretty violent. These students, unfortunately, weren't considering their larger environment. They blatantly stood out as easy marks compared with the locals.

While we all want to stand out at times and get noticed, there are other times when it's smarter to try to blend in with the crowd, using your body language, clothes, and nonverbal communication.

Now that we've covered how to use your body language to protect yourself from predators, let's talk about reading other people's body language. How do you identify hostile people through their body language?

That's what we'll discover in the next chapter.

Important Points:

- ◊ Body language and nonverbal communication is very important; experts estimate that up to 93 percent of all communication is nonverbal.

- ◊ There are three key rules of body language:
    1. Read body language in clusters.
    2. Consider the context of the situation.
    3. Consider the culture of the person whom you are studying.

- ◊ Body language awareness can be used from everything from the boardroom to the bedroom.

- ◊ What message are you sending to others on a daily basis? If you want to change the results you're getting, consider looking at your nonverbal cues.

- ◊ You can use body language and nonverbal signals to 'fail' a predator interview and avoid becoming a victim.

- ◊ Common suggestions include direct eye contact, standing up straight, projecting confidence, relaying an awareness of your situation, and squarely facing your opponent.

- ◊ It's also important to consider your dress and what messages your clothes are sending about you.

- ◊ When facing new situations—and potentially dangerous situations—there is merit in not standing out and in trying to blend in.

Body Language Exercise:

#1: Take a week and consciously work on your body language. Try to project a stronger (not tougher) energy. Stand up taller. Show your awareness of your situation. Walk confidently.

Notice how people treat you. Do they treat you differently? With more respect? How do you see yourself? Does your body language affect the way you feel?

#2: Now take a week (or a few days) and practice showing weak body language: quiet voice, hunched shoulders, downward gaze. See how people treat you. Do they treat you differently?

How do you feel about yourself? Does your body language affect the way you feel in this situation?

 # 3: Take some time and consider what image you're currently projecting to others. If you're feeling really brave, ask some good friends what kind of image and energy you project to them.

Now ask yourself if this is in line with what you want to project. If not, what kind of image do you want to project, and what steps will it take to get you there?

Chapter 10 –
What Are Other People Telling You? Reading Others' Hidden Intentions through Their Body Language

By Chuck O'Neill

"When the eyes say one thing, and the tongue another, a practiced man relies on the language of the first." — Ralph Waldo Emerson

Lorelai: "Well, what was his body language like?"
Rory: "Tall."
— Gilmore Girls

In the last chapter you learned several ways to use your own body language to protect yourself. But what about reading other people? How do you use body language and nonverbal communication to discover what others are really saying?

First of all, I have great news for you: Most people, yourself included, are actually very good at reading body language. You were born with the skill to read other people's nonverbal signals.

After all, that's how you knew you were in trouble when Mom gave you 'the look' as a kid. That's how you figured out that the girl who smiled at you in class might actually like you. That's how you sensed that the coworker leaning in a little too close might be hitting on you.

So the good news is that you already have an inherent skill to read others' intentions. The bad news is that you probably don't use it.

In fact, because of our highly independent, computerized, social-media-replacing-real-social-contact lifestyles, I'd estimate that probably 90 percent of people today don't use this innate skill. And just like any skill set, it will get rusty with disuse. But you can develop it again with practice and with what you'll learn in this chapter.

Before long, you'll start to pick up on things you never noticed before, like the woman who gets nervous every time you mention her boyfriend or the salesman who shows signs of hostility over a certain part of the sales contract or the politician who is lying about having sex with that woman.

The Fundamentals of Reading Other People's Body Language:

Recall the three key fundamentals about body language we covered in the previous chapter. They still apply here as well:

1. **Read body language in clusters.**
2. **Consider the context of the situation.**
3. **Consider the culture of the person whom you are studying.**

There is one more fundamental when it comes to reading other people:

#4: You must establish a baseline (if possible): While there are certain universal signals that tend to mean the same thing (e.g., excessive blinking or touching face when lying, shaking head in disagreement, crossing arms when in disagreement, etc.), you still must consider the baseline of the person that you're observing.

The baseline is basically the way the person acts on a regular basis, and it's unique for everyone. By keeping this baseline in mind, it's much easier to spot when that person may become a danger to themselves or to you because they will vary from their baseline.

Here's the bottom line: When someone varies widely from their baseline, it's worth investigating further.

For instance, let's say that in your capacity as a social worker, you come in contact with a client named John, who is on medication for schizophrenia. You know from experience with John that, while on his proper medication, he tends to be pretty calm. He's quiet, friendly, open, and usually pretty responsive to your suggestions.

That's his baseline.

Now let's say that one day you meet with John and he is not smiling. He's jumpy; restless; making grandiose, nonsensical statements; and refusing to make eye contact with you.

From this situation—and knowing John's baseline—you can tell that something's wrong. Perhaps his medication is off. Maybe something devastating just happened to him. Regardless, it's worth investigating further.

As another example, let's say you worked in your office with a young man named Dave. Dave is a bit of a hothead. He's very social and is always planning a company softball game, Super Bowl party, or office get-together with plenty of alcohol. He likes to talk—a lot. You know everything about Dave because he's told you everything. There seems to be virtually no filter on his mouth; he has a bad case of verbal diarrhea.

Now let's say that you come into the office one Monday morning expecting Dave to come and give you the usual rundown of his weekend activities. Instead, Dave stays in his office. There's no knock on your door, no jovial smile as he plunks down in the chair and sloshes his coffee cup down on your desk. In fact, you start to wonder if Dave might be sick.

You stop by his office and he barely looks up from his desk.

"Hey, buddy," you say. "How was your weekend?"

"Fine," is all the response he gives you.

Shrugging, you go on your way, secretly grateful for the reprieve from Dave's weekend adventure stories. You might actually get some work done this morning.

But throughout the week, Dave continues to stick to his office, keeping his nose in his work. He doesn't mention any parties. He doesn't try out his latest in-very-poor-taste joke on the new office secretary. He doesn't even suggest a drink after work to anyone. This happens the next week as well—no more jovial, back-slapping Dave telling highly inappropriate jokes to the office crowd.

This would probably be the time where you'll want to investigate. Dave is deviating from a well-established baseline. He's performing actions that would be normal for other people (staying in his office, doing his work, not being overly sociable). But in Dave's case, it's a huge deviation from his personal baseline.

What could have happened?

Any number of things. Dave could have broken up with his girlfriend or lost a close family member. He could now be struggling with depression.

Dave could have heard a rumor that he was going to lose his job and is now trying to decide whether he should sabotage the company in some way.

Or he could have just been diagnosed with a serious cancer and he's struggling to deal with the physical and emotional fallout.

The important thing is that this is a red flag because he's not acting in line with his baseline (even though it would be considered normal behavior for other people). It would be smart in this situation to investigate further.

When people deviate from their baseline, it should tell you something.

Kate and I bought a house several years back in North Toronto. While we loved the house, the seller was a nightmare. We went back and forth negotiating. He was petty and mean. He didn't want to budge on anything.

He complained to his agent throughout the entire process (which we heard about from our agent). He gave no concessions. He even ended up taking the central vac attachments and bolted-on mirrors from all five bathrooms when he left. (And no, they were not part of the contract!)

That, unfortunately, was his baseline.

He was even true to form on the day we moved in. He took all day to move out. (He was supposed to be gone by 5 p.m.). By 7 p.m. he was still there, casually joking with the movers as they struggled to finish their job.

After a long day of moving out of our old house and three hours of waiting outside our new house in an uncomfortably warm moving van, Kate had reached her boiling point. She marched into the house, much to the seller's surprise, and faced him down as only a feisty, fed-up, redhead can do. She then announced that she couldn't wait for him any longer and started to clean.

Then something odd happened—he was nice to her. He started telling her what a great house it was and how we were going to enjoy living there.

As it was summer, he started explaining in detail how, with the proper opening of certain windows, we could get a great cross breeze through the house. Doing it this way, he explained, meant we wouldn't have to use the air conditioning, which would save us money. Kate was flattered and figured that it was her natural charm that made the seller so magnanimous.

I had my doubts, however. This was a huge deviation from his baseline, and my gut told me something was off.

Unfortunately, we found out a week later that I was right. How? We turned on the air conditioning, and it didn't work.

We had followed the seller's advice to keep the windows open for a week, but, with a sudden heat spike, we decided to close the windows and try the air conditioning instead. Nothing. It was completely dead—in the middle of one of the hottest summers we'd had in years. And because we hadn't tested it out the day we moved in, we had no recourse to go back to the seller and get him to pay for the broken air conditioning unit.

We ended up with an $800 repair bill and a repair guy who told us that the unit had probably been broken for months.

The seller's sudden charm had to do with the fact that he didn't want us to try out the air conditioning unit on the day of closing so that we couldn't make him pay for the repairs. (When you buy a house, you're supposed to test everything on closing day to make sure it's in good working order so that you can go back to the seller and make them pay for it if it's not.)

We should have noticed the red flag when the seller deviated from his baseline by acting cordial and friendly when he had only been surly and difficult up to that point in time.

So it's important to pay attention to somebody's baseline when possible. When you notice deviations—in body language or actions—it's a sure sign that something is off.

How to Identify Hostile Body Language:

How do you know when someone is feeling hostile towards you? How do you know when they're about to go off on you or set a trap for you?

Reading their body language can help expose their intensions. Here are some common signals of hostile body language:

#1: Crossing Your Boundaries without an Invitation: When people cross your boundaries, physical or emotional, without invitation, it can be seen as a hostile or controlling act. (We're going to talk more about boundaries in another chapter, but this ties in with body language as well.)

For example, if someone is leaning in closer to you than is polite, they are invading your boundaries, which may actually be a hostile action. Other ways they might cross your boundaries are claiming your things—like your food, your space, or your personal items.

They may make inappropriate sexual jokes or make assumptions for you as to what you'll have to eat or how long you're going to stay at their home. They may physically touch you when you clearly are not asking for it, and ignore your request for them to stop.

Any time somebody is crossing your boundaries—physical or emotional—it is a hostile action. It indicates they may be trying to control you. If you continue to let them, this could escalate into a confrontation.

#2: Generally Hostile Body Language: There are certain signs that are generally acknowledged universally as hostile actions.

Some of these are:

◊ crossing the arms across the chest

◊ leaning away from a person

◊ frowning

◊ narrowing the eyes

◊ tightening and/or pursing of the lips

◊ angling the body away from another person

- ◊ turning your feet away from the person or crossing your legs away from the person

- ◊ smiling with your mouth only (the smile doesn't 'reach your eyes')

- ◊ breaking eye contact or refusing to establish eye contact

- ◊ limp hand shake or making sure their hand is on top of yours (a sign of dominance)

- ◊ snorting in response to a comment

- ◊ shaking the head back and forth (saying 'no' with your head)

- ◊ flaring of the nostrils

- ◊ showing disrespect in your dress (e.g., an entrepreneur dressing in jeans and a hoodie to pitch his latest idea to a potential millionaire investor)

These are all generally hostile signs that you can look for (in clusters) when assessing if someone feels hostile towards you.

That's not to say they will attack you. Depending on the situation, they may just turn down your proposal, not give you that job, or slander your character behind your back. Again, it depends on the situation and what is at stake.

#3: Physical Actions That Don't Match Their Words: When people's actions don't match their words (also called incongruence), that can be a hostile sign or a sign that you're being lied to.

For example, I recently watched Oprah interview the now-disgraced cyclist Lance Armstrong. This man is known to have cheated and lied for years about doping in his sport. While I found the entire interview a fascinating study in hostile body language, I was particularly struck by how many times his actions did not match his words.

For example, when he made an affirmative statement that he deserved the punishment that he got, he shook his head back and forth (in a 'no' gesture). This showed—to me at least—that he didn't really think he deserved his punishment.

When he denied an allegation, saying it wasn't true, he actually nodded his head in the affirmative (saying with his body language that it was true). This was a clear display of actions not matching words. And it can be a sign of hostility, lying, or both.

A lot of us guys experience this action-word mismatch on a more harmless level with our significant others. As guys we can be lunkheads sometimes. And I always know when I've been particularly lunkheaded because my wife's actions won't match her words.

How many times, guys, have you lived through a conversation like this:

"Honey, is something wrong?"

"No—nothing's wrong." (This is said with a cold dispassion that you KNOW is not her usual tone.)

"Are you sure? Did I do something?"

"Nope. Nothing."

Okay, at this point she's probably turning away, not looking at you, not touching you, and you're still being a lunkhead, not realizing the words don't match the actions. You might make a final attempt here.

"Are you sure? You seem upset."

"Why should I be upset?"

Now guys, this is not an invitation to shrug your shoulders and go on your merry way. This is a question you should think long and hard about answering. Because I guarantee you, if you don't get the answer right, you're in for a world of hurt.

This is a great example of the fact that her words and actions are not matching up, so somewhere along the line you probably screwed up. And she's now feeling pretty hostile towards you.

Now contrast this with what you would feel if this conversation happened and she was still snuggling up to you and using that adoring tone you love so much:

"Honey, is something wrong?"

"No, nothing's wrong." (This is said as she rubs your chest and kisses your cheek.)

"Are you sure? Did I do something?"

"Nope, nothing." She shakes her head and then grins at you.

That conversation takes on a whole other meaning, doesn't it?

Why?

Because her words and actions matched up.

(If more of us guys could get this one simple principle, we'd all be a whole lot happier.)

#4: Flashes of Hostility: In point #2 we talked about general, large, sweeping signs of hostility. However, there can also be smaller flashes of hostility that are harder to pick up—but not impossible.

For example, the quick smirk just before a narcissist lies to you gives you a clue that they feel superior enough to pull the wool over your eyes.

#5: Signs of Lying: We're going to cover this more fully in the next chapter, but it applies here as well. There are many small signals of insincerity you can learn to see if someone is lying to you.

For example, many experts say that liars tend to blink more than usual when telling a fib. Another common sign is the constant touching of the face (which is an unconscious attempt to cover the mouth and hide the lie coming out of it).

In certain circumstances, a person pausing before answering your question may indicate lying. (It could also indicate trying to recall a memory, so be careful here.)

I once had a cop friend of mine tell me that one of the biggest signs someone is lying is that they repeat your question.

"Do you have drugs in your car?"

"Are you asking me if I have drugs in this car, officer?"

By repeating your question, they are trying to give themselves time to come up with a believable answer.

Other signs of liars are people who give too many details in their answers, details you never asked for like:

"Did you take the money in my wallet?"

"Why would I take the money in your wallet? I just got $80 from Dad to buy that new dress I told you about, the one with the pink flowers on it. I'm going to the mall this afternoon to get it."

In this situation a simple 'No' would have been the honest answer, or even "No—why would I do that?" By adding too many details, the person is trying too hard to convince the other person of their honesty.

Another sign of a liar is someone who doesn't give a direct answer to a simple question. For example:

"Did you sue her?"

"You know, we sued so many people it's hard to keep track."

Again, this isn't saying that the person is straight-out lying, but you should be asking yourself why they're trying so hard to avoid giving you a simple, straight answer.

#6: Behaviors That Don't Fit: Remember how we talked about being aware of things that didn't fit? You can use this in body language as well.

For example, let's say you pull into a parking lot to visit a bank machine. The parking lot is fairly empty except for one guy who doesn't seem to be doing much of anything. There's no car. He hasn't just come from the bank machine. He's standing alone, maybe on a cell phone, and he's wandering closer to your car while talking on his phone.

This might be a red flag because it's a behavior that doesn't fit what you'd usually see in that situation.

Or let's say you're shopping in a lingerie store and you notice a man watching you intently. He isn't looking at the bras, and he isn't asking a sales girl for help to find something for his girlfriend. He's watching you.

What doesn't fit here?

I once had a couple of girls approach me in a parking lot asking for change. They claimed they'd locked their cell phones and purses in their car and couldn't get to them, so they needed change for the bus to get home. They even told me I could come with them to see their car to prove their story.

There were a few things that didn't fit here.

First of all, this was a well-known, fairly affluent mall in South Florida; they even had mall security cars going up and down the aisles to make sure people were okay, giving rides to people with heavy bags, etc.

So surely these girls could have gotten the security officers to help them get into their car or even call a locksmith and pay him once they got to their purses.

These girls were well dressed, which means they clearly were not homeless. What teenage girl can't call her parents collect and ask to be picked up at the mall? It's practically a rite of passage as a teenager to call home because you've locked your keys in your car.

Then there was their offer to take me to their car to prove their story. This goes to the lying issue we talked about above. They were trying too hard to prove to me that their story was legit, which means it probably wasn't.

And why ask for money for the bus of all things? Why not stop people and ask if they know how to get into a locked car? Why not ask if you can borrow a cell phone to call your parents, a friend, or even AAA?

Finally, these girls were also acting smug, almost flirtatious with me. What teenage girl acts coy and cute when she's just locked her keys in her car? Most girls in that situation would probably be panicked, upset, and sincerely asking people for help—most likely the security staff at the mall, not total strangers in a parking lot.

These girls were definitely displaying behaviors that didn't fit the situation (or at least the situation as they told it). I decided to pass and told them I had no change (which I didn't).

They moved on to the next gentlemen walking to his car. I'll never know what the real story was, but I do know that something was off.

And in reality, that's all you really need to know to stay safe. When something seems like it doesn't fit, move on.

Specific Body Language Immediately before Physical Hostility

What about if you're concerned about a physical altercation? How can you tell if someone is going to lunge for you?

There are also several specific body signs that people tend to display before they attack you physically. They are:

#1: The Fist Pump: This is when you're in a heated argument with a guy and you notice he's making a fist and releasing it over and over again. When he stops pumping and the argument continues to escalate, that could be a sign that he's getting ready to hit you. (People need a split second to build up to the action of hitting you.)

#2: The "Ready to Spring" Position: If you're talking with someone and they have their legs crossed or stretched out in front of them, they're probably not a threat at that moment. It's when they're sitting with both feet flat on the floor, on the balls of the feet, and slightly leaning forward that they may be getting ready to spring at you.

#3: Turning the Body to Hide a Weapon: If you approach someone and they specifically turn away from you to hide one side of their body (usually the right side, where a knife or gun might be located), that's a red flag. They may be trying to hide a weapon from you.

This has also been used when people are in arguments. They start off square, facing each other, then for no reason one person turns away slightly and goes into a semi-submissive state then cold cocks the other person.

In another vein, they may also try to hide a weapon by untucking or rearranging their shirt over the weapon.

#4: The Index Finger Jab: Nobody likes it when someone waves their index finger at them. But when the index-finger-waving motion transforms into an index-finger-jabbing motion, it can quickly turn into a fist jabbing—straight at your face.

#5: Crossing into Your Personal Space: When someone is purposely violating your personal space (or getting "all up in your grill"), it can very easily lead to a physical attack. They've already crossed one boundary by violating your personal space. It's very easy to cross the next logical boundary and hit you as things escalate.

#6: The Thumb Twitch: When you see the thumb twitch upwards, you may have a split second before your attacker reaches for his gun or knife.

Predators who are planning to go for their gun will often raise their thumb up in anticipation of going for their weapon. (They will need to raise their thumb to get their weapon out of the holster.)

So those are some common signs of hostile body language that can occur right before an attack. When you're in a yellow or red zone alert situation, keep an eye out for these signs and take steps to protect yourself if you see them happening.

Now, not all hostile acts are physical; sometimes people just want to manipulate you, con you, and steal from you. In those cases they will probably lie to you.

How can you spot a liar? That's what you'll discover in the next chapter.

Important Points:

◊ One of the most important rules of reading other people's body language is to establish a baseline. Anything that differs from that person's norm may be worth investigating.

◊ Common signs of hostile body language include crossing the arms, lying, frowning, closed body positioning, flashes of hostility, words that don't match actions, and behaviors that don't fit the situation.

◊ Common signs of a pending physical attack are the fist pump, the jabbing finger, violating your personal space, the thumb twitch, and getting ready to spring.

◊ When you spot hostile body language, depending on the situation, either seek to remove yourself or put up boundaries to protect yourself.

Body Language Exercise – Reading Hostile Intentions

#1: Take a few hours and go to a heavily trafficked area like a mall or a food court area. Watch other people for signs of hostile body language. How many can you pick up? What are the most common signs of hostile body language that you see?

#2: Practice looking for incongruence in body language. For example, does the waiter smile but it doesn't reach his eyes? Does your boss cross his arms and shake his head while telling you that he likes your idea?

#3: Watch celebrity interviews, or go to YouTube and look up past celebrity interviews like Lance Armstrong's with Oprah or Bill Clinton being questioned about Monica Lewinsky. See if you can spot any hostile body language signs.

Chapter 11 –
How to Be a Human Lie Detector – Body Language and Verbal Tells

By Kate O'Neill

> *"If you tell the truth, you don't have to remember anything."*
> — Mark Twain

> *"When it comes to controlling human beings there is no better instrument than lies. Because, you see, humans live by beliefs. And beliefs can be manipulated. The power to manipulate beliefs is the only thing that counts."* — Michael Ende, The Neverending Story

Can you tell when someone is lying to you? Do you know the signs to look for?

There are entire books devoted solely to being able to detect liars and the lies they tell. You'll find some of the best ones listed in Appendix A of this book. However, if you don't want to make a life study out of it, this chapter will give you some of the key points to know about how to tell when people are lying to you.

We're not talking here about the occasional white lie people tell to grease the wheels of polite social conversation. That's normal. Everybody lies from time to time. If we told people what we really thought of them sometimes, none of us would be speaking to each other.

We're talking here about spotting the person who is lying to you as an act of aggression. We're talking about the person who lies in order to manipulate, con, and steal from you.

Being able to spot these people is just one more skill you can use in your arsenal for psychological self-defense.

The first thing you should know about spotting a liar is that it's not an exact science. Just like reading body language, you have to look for clusters of behavior.

You can't just say, "See, he's touching his nose a lot; that means he's lying." Or "She's giving too many details, so she must be lying." You have to take into account the whole picture, the situation around you, and the baseline of that specific person. (Recall that the baseline is what is normal for that specific person.)

So even though you're going to learn some common signs that someone is lying to you, keep in mind you must look for clusters of behavior to confirm your hypothesis.

Body Language Tells vs. Verbal Tells

There are two basic groups of behaviors to look at when spotting a lie. The first is the person's body language—what they do before, during, and after they lie. The second group is the common verbal tells that liars display.

I've personally found that detecting lies based on somebody's verbal tells tends to be more reliable. Body language can be much less precise but still very useful. And when you become skilled enough to use them together, it's a very powerful skill set indeed.

Let's start with body language.

Common Body Language Signs of Liars

#1: Action-Word Disconnect: We touched on this a bit in the Body Language chapter. This is when you see a disconnect between what somebody is saying and what they are doing. (This is also called congruency in some body language circles—you're looking for the words and actions to match.)

For example, if you ask Sarah if she took the cookies on the counter and she nods her head up and down while saying, "Mom, I NEVER took the cookies!" that is a disconnect.

If you're pitching an idea to your boss and your boss says, "Go ahead, I'm open to new ideas," but he has his arms folded, his legs crossed, and his chin down, that's a disconnect.

Joe Navarro, in his book *What Every BODY is Saying*, tells the story about being called in to interview a suspect in a rape case. The suspect claimed he was walking past the field where the rape occurred on his way home. He said he had turned right to go home, which took him away from the field. However, Joe noticed that as he said this, the suspect gestured to the left—the exact way he would have gone to get to the scene of the crime.

Because Joe caught that one small gesture that didn't agree with the suspect's words, he was able to investigate further and find out that the suspect had indeed committed the rape.

#2: Touching the Face / Covering the Mouth: This gesture goes back to when we were young and had the childish impulse to cover the mouth when we knew that what was coming out of it was not true. When children lie, they often cover their mouths, which is a dead giveaway for parents.

However, we get a little more sophisticated as we get older. We may cover our mouths in a speculative gesture (e.g., thumb and forefinger touching the mouth). We may also touch our nose, scratch our chin, or wipe our forehead.

Note, however, that this gesture can also indicate the speaker is holding something back or feeling anxious or uncertain about what he's saying (not necessarily lying).

"The original Mouth-Covering gesture becomes even faster in adulthood. When an adult tells a lie, it's as if his brain instructs his hand to cover his mouth in an attempt to block the deceitful words, just as it did for the five-year-old and the teenager.

But, at the last moment the hand is pulled away from the face and a Nose-Touch gesture results. This is simply an adult's version of the Mouth-Covering gesture that was used in childhood." — Allan and Barbara Pease, *The Definitive Book of Body Language*

#3: Rubbing the Eyes: Someone who is lying may attempt to block out their deceitful words by rubbing their eyes. They may also just rub the area around their eyes (to the side or just below). This is an unconscious attempt to block out the lie (a form of 'see no evil').

#4: Touching the Neck or Ears: Again, this may be a subverted form of covering the mouth or eyes like in #3 above. It can also be a self-soothing gesture as the person is anxious about telling the lie.

For example, women often reach up to play with a necklace or play with the neck clavicle area in an attempt to self-soothe. They may be anxious about lying, but they could also be anxious because they feel vulnerable with the topic of conversation.

#5: Blinking Excessively: Many experts claim that people tend to blink excessively when they are being untruthful. For example, it's been reported that when Bill Clinton gave his 1998 speech to the nation about the Monica Lewinsky scandal, he blinked about 120 times per minute.

Normally, we blink about 15 to 30 times per minute and up to 50 times per minute when in front of a camera). When someone appears to be blinking more than that, it could be a sign of discomfort or anxiety, possibly because they are being untruthful.

#6: Excessive Fidgeting and Gesturing: When people lie, they get anxious because they know they're doing something wrong. This comes out in a number of ways; one of these may be through excessive fidgeting and gesturing. They may play with the coffee cup in front of them or tap their feet under the table.

Again, however, this could also be a result of anxiety for a different reason. They could be bored. They could be worried about a situation at work. Or they may have just had an extra shot of espresso that morning.

#7: Looking away from You or at You, Intensely: Many people think that when someone looks away from you, they're lying. And sometimes this is true; a liar may avert his gaze from you at the point where he starts to tell his lie.

However, scientists have also found that some liars may actually maintain better eye contact when they are lying to you (perhaps as a way to convince you of their sincerity).So you may notice someone looking at you a bit too intensely when fibbing.

Another thing they may do is to look down. Studies have shown that we tend to look up (and to the right) when we are trying to recall memories (truthful information). But we look down when we're accessing our imagination (to make things up).

#8: Micro Gestures: Micro gestures are tiny, fleeting movements that are hard to spot for most people. But they can often leak out when someone is lying.

For example, I recently watched an interview of a famous celebrity who was apologizing for verbally attacking a woman who had accused him of wrongdoing.

As he expressed his 'sincere' regret at attacking the woman, he let slip a small, very fleeting sneer. It was hard to catch, but it was definitely there. This (along with a few other signs) showed me that the man probably wasn't sorry he'd attacked this woman at all. His real attitude towards her was haughty and hateful.

Micro gestures can be so hard to catch that many times body language experts have to watch a video frame by frame to catch them. For that reason, I don't put a lot of stock in them because most people won't be able to catch them unless trained to do so.

#9: Hiding Hands or Moving away from You: For most people, gesturing with their palms open is a sign of sincerity. ("See? I've got nothing to hide from you.") On the flip side of this coin, however, you may notice that a liar wants to hide his hands from you or even hide his whole body by unconsciously moving away from you.

#10: Slight Shoulder Shrug: If someone is lying, or just unsure of what they're saying, you may notice a slight shoulder shrug—either both shoulders or one side only. Shrugging your shoulders is a signal of uncertainty; you're basically saying, "I don't know."

So when someone does this—even subtly—while saying something in the affirmative that they SHOULD know, it can be a sign you may want to investigate.

For example, a few years ago, a friend of mine was dating a guy she was pretty serious about. I got the chance to speak to him at a social gathering. Knowing she was a good friend of mine, in the course of our conversation (and probably trying to convince me), he said, "Yup, I know this is it. She's the girl for me."

This was followed, however, by a very subtle right shoulder shrug. I suspected then that he wasn't really sure of his feelings at all. Unfortunately, a week later, the guy told my friend he wasn't ready for a commitment and broke up with her. His true feelings had been there all along in his body language the night we spoke.

Common Verbal Tells Liars Use

So those are some common body language clues to look for when someone might be lying to you. Body language clues can be invaluable in helping you to spot a liar. However, you always have to keep in mind the person's baseline, the situation, and the circumstances around you.

For this reason, I've found that the most reliable lie-detector signals actually come from the actual mouths of the liars themselves—the verbal tells.

And if you're not very good at picking up on body language— or if you're just more of an auditory person than a visual person— it might be easier to analyze the words a person says to look for signs of lying.

> *"Resist the urge to fill in missing information when listening to a person's story. Pay attention to exactly what is said and not said"*
> *— Pamela Meyer, Proven Techniques to Detect Deception*

Here are some common verbal 'tells' that liars commonly display:

#1: Using Phrases like "Honestly," "To Tell the Truth," and "Truth Be Told": While it may seem ironic, liars tend to use phrases like, "I have to be honest with you...," "Truthfully...," "Honestly...," and other honesty reinforcements. They need these reinforcements because they are trying doubly hard to convince you of their lie. If they were telling the truth, they wouldn't have to reinforce it with an honesty phrase.

Now sometimes people just use these phrases for extra dramatic emphasis, and sometimes they may just be exaggerating.

However, why would someone have to add the 'Honestly' to their sentence? Wouldn't you assume that what they are saying was truthful in the first place?

#2: They Use Qualifiers: Similar to the honesty reinforcers above, liars will also use qualifiers like "To the best of my knowledge," "As far as I know," and "I could be wrong but...." By using these qualifiers, they're basically covering their you-know-what.

And you have to ask yourself, if they know what they're saying is true, why do they have to couch it like that?

Do you say to your wife, "To the best of my knowledge, I've never cheated on you"? Do you say to your boss, "I could be wrong, but I don't think I've ever stolen money from the company"?

No. Because you know.

When I hear people use wishy-washy qualifiers (celebrities or politicians caught in scandals are famous for this), I'm always suspicious of what they're saying.

#3: They Don't Give You Straight Answers to Simple Questions: This is one of the easiest verbal tells of a liar. They won't give you a straight answer. They'll dance around and try to distract you, but it will seem virtually impossible to get them to just give you a 'no' or a 'yes' answer.

If you ask them, for example, "Did you take the money on my dresser?" they may say,

"Why would I take money from your dresser? Why would I do something like that? You know I have my own money that I earned from babysitting last week."

Notice that you never actually got an answer to your question?

Years ago, I read about a man accused of killing his girlfriend and burying her body in the backyard. He denied it at first. This is what he said when they questioned him:

Officer: "Did you kill your girlfriend?"

Suspect: "I never hurt my girlfriend. I love her. I would never hurt my girlfriend."

Notice that he didn't actually answer the question?

He denied hurting his girlfriend—but not killing her. He went on to later admit that he had indeed killed his girlfriend and buried her in his backyard.

#4: Repeating Your Question: Recall from the last chapter the police officer who said that the number one way he knows a suspect is lying is when he repeats his questions back to him:

"Do you have drugs in your car?"

"Officer, are you asking me if I have drugs in my car?"

"Are you carrying a knife?"

"Am I carrying a knife—is that what you're asking me?"

This repeating of the question is a common tactic to allow the liar time to come up with a good lie that he thinks you'll believe.

#5: Commenting on Your Question: This is similar to #4 in that the person is buying time to respond in a way he thinks you'll believe. So for example, someone might say something like "That's a good question..." or "I'm glad you asked that because...."

Sometimes, if the person is really good, they can turn that opening comment on your question into a distraction and manage to avoid answering the question altogether.

For example, "I'm glad you asked that question—because so many people are asking the wrong questions here. What I really want to focus on is the issue behind this, which is women's rights...."

They never actually get around to answering the question but instead were able to segue into another issue to distract from the original question.

#6: Attacking the Questioner: This is a common tactic that a liar uses—especially if they feel threatened—to get the questioner to back off. They may turn around and make you feel guilty for attacking them.

You may hear things like, "Who do you think you are anyway?" "What's your problem? Why can't you let it go?" or "Why are you attacking me this way?" (thereby attacking you by accusing you of attacking them).

"Being backed into a corner by the facts of a situation can put a lot of strain on a deceptive person and can compel him to go on the attack. This might take the form of an attempt to impeach your credibility or competence. ... What he's trying to do is to get you to back off, to start questioning yourself on whether you're going down the right path."
—Philip Houston, Michael Floyd, and Susan Carnicero, Spy the Lie

#7: Convincing Statements: These take on the form of describing who this person is in order to convince you they would never do anything like that.

They might say, "I've worked for this company for twenty years; I would never put my job at risk," or "I'm an honest person; I would never lie," or even "I believe in the sanctity of marriage; I would never violate it by cheating."

For example, in Lance Armstrong's 2005 sworn deposition, he was asked if he had ever taken performance-enhancing drugs. He used several convincing statements like this one:

> *"If you have a doping offense or you test positive, it goes without saying that you're fired from all of your contracts, not just the team, but there's [touching his nose] numerous contracts that I have that would all go away ... and*

the faith of all the cancer survivors around the world, so everything I do off of the bike would go away, too ... and don't think for a second that I don't understand that ...

it's also about the faith that people have put in me over the years, so all of that would be erased. So I don't need it to say in a contract 'you're fired if you test positive.' That's not as important as losing the support of hundreds of millions of people."

Pretty convincing, right?

Convincing statements can be very effective because they sound so good. They say in effect, "Look at me. I'm such a good person. I would obviously NEVER do something like that."

But when someone is trying to convince you of their goodness instead of just answering your question, it can be a red flag that they're lying.

"The more he talked of his honour the faster we counted our spoons."
    — *Ralph Waldo Emerson*

#8: Pausing before Answering: This is a sign of lying only in certain circumstances. For example, if you ask a question that a person should know the answer to right away and they pause, that's a bad sign.

But if you ask them something they should have to think about to remember, that is not a sign of lying. (Consequently, if they answer too fast in this situation, it may be something to worry about.)

For example, if you ask somebody, "Have you ever cheated on your wife?" and they pause to think about it, that's a bad sign. They should be able to answer immediately 'No.'

On the other hand, if you ask someone, "What did you have for dinner last Saturday?" they'll probably need to pause and think about it.

It also depends on the specific person's situation.

For example, if you ask your friend, "Did you see Larry last Tuesday?" and they see Larry several times a week, they may have to pause and think about it. They'll have to access their memory to see if Tuesday was a day that they did, in fact, see Larry.

If, however, they haven't seen Larry in ten years, they won't have to pause to think about whether or not they saw him last week because it will stand out in their minds.

#9: Giving Too Many Details: If someone gives you too many details, especially details that you never asked for, it can be a sign that they're lying. They're trying too hard to convince you.

For example, when I worked at a bank some years back, a man came in to apply for a second mortgage on his house. While many people are nervous in a loan application interview, I noticed that this man seemed much more nervous than usual.

Why? He was talking too much, telling me about his job and what repairs (in detail) he planned to do on the house. I never asked him these things, but he automatically told me about them—which made me suspicious. He was clearly too nervous.

When I investigated a little further, I found out my suspicions were right. The house was actually owned by both the man and his wife. After making a few calls, I found out the man and his wife had recently decided to get a divorce.

The wife had no idea the man was trying to take out money from the house with a second mortgage. He was trying to get it without her knowing and without disclosing this information to the bank.

#10: Giving Overly Vague Answers: When someone lies—especially on the fly—they don't have time to think of the details. So you'll probably get vague answers like, "Oh I had some errands to run," or "She said something bad about you—I can't remember what it was."

That doesn't mean that one vague answer is a lie, but again, look for clusters. And also try questioning them further. If they still avoid giving you details, it can be a red flag.

#11: Distancing Themselves: When someone lies, they unconsciously want to distance themselves from the situation they are lying about. This can take the form of using proper names. It can also take the form of using full words vs. normal contractions (e.g., they are vs. they're; you are vs. you're).

Bill Clinton did this when he famously lied to the press about Monica Lewinsky:

"I did not have sexual relations with that woman—Miss Lewinsky."

Notice the 'did not' vs. 'didn't' and 'that woman—Miss Lewinsky' vs. 'Monica Lewinsky.'

Sometimes It's Not What They Say; It's What They *Don't* Say

Sometimes it's not what a person is saying to you that alerts you to the lie; it's what they don't say. You have to ask yourself if their reaction was normal given the specific situation.

Take the example of Susan Smith, the woman who drowned her two young boys in 1995 and then lied about it, saying the boys were taken by a carjacker.

When she went on television with a plea to the 'carjacker' to give her boys back, she showed several signs of lying. These signs included speaking about her boys in the past tense as if they were already dead ("my children needed me"), looking down, and shading her eyes by keeping her eyelids almost closed.

However, the big giveaway for many was what she *didn't* show. Her crying was forced. She didn't display the emotion that a normal mother who'd just lost her kids would show. There was no tenseness in her face, no wrinkled forehead, no tears or clenched jaw.

Contrast that with her husband who spoke to the cameras a moment later and you saw the difference.

He was trying with everything he had to hold it together. His face was tight, his forehead wrinkled. His jaw was clenched tightly in a bid to keep control. He was showing genuine emotion—emotion that reached out and touched everyone who watched.

How to Handle a Liar

So what can you do when you think someone is lying to you? One thing I advise people is to avoid going for the direct confrontation. If someone knows you're onto them, they may just become more firmly entrenched in their lie. Or they may clam up altogether.

Try coming at them from the side. Keep them talking; the more they talk, the more they are likely to reveal inconsistencies in their story—if they are truly lying. Ask them questions, but try not to be obvious about it.

Another thing you can do is investigate their claims further if you can. See if you can verify what that person is saying.

If they say they've worked at a certain company, call the company or go to their website to verify. If they say that somebody said something about you, call up that person and ask them if they said that thing about you. (Now, this person could be lying too, but at least you're going straight to the source.)

Verify in any way you can. And when you find evidence of lying, you'll have a good idea of this person's character. You'll know that you can't trust what they tell you in the future. You may even choose to cut them out of your life, depending on how toxic they are.

If you can't cut them out of your life, you may also want to put up boundaries to protect yourself. We're going to cover how you can do this in the next chapter.

Important Points:

- ◊ Everybody lies, but when someone is lying repeatedly to you in order to manipulate, con, or take from you, it is an act of aggression and you must protect yourself.
- ◊ Spotting a liar is not an exact science as there are some very good liars out there (and some poor ones, too).
- ◊ There is no one definite sign that proves someone is lying to you. You have to look at clusters of behavior within the context of the situation.
- ◊ Liars give themselves away (usually numerous times) in both body language and verbal tells.
- ◊ Common body language signs of lying are covering the mouth, touching the face or nose, fidgeting, excessive blinking, looking away from you, hiding the hands, or turning the body away while still facing you.
- ◊ Common verbal tells of liars include using honesty reinforcing statements, convincing statements, qualifiers, giving too many details, repeating the question, and pausing before answering.
- ◊ Look also for what they may not be saying (that they should be). For example, is this a natural reaction given the circumstances?
- ◊ If you think someone is lying to you, try to find out more information from them without being obvious about it. Try to verify the truth of their statements.

◊ When you know someone has repeatedly lied to you, don't take it lightly. They've proven they're not trustworthy and don't have your best interests at heart. Take steps to protect yourself.

How to Spot a Liar Exercise

Practice spotting a liar. Go to YouTube and look up interviews from celebrities who are known to have lied to the press (e.g., the Lance Armstrong 2005 doping interview, Bill Clinton's testimony on Monika Lewinsky, Anthony Wiener and the sexting scandal, Marion Jones's CBS denial about steroid use, Richard Nixon's 'I'm Not a Crook' speech).

Watch for the body language and verbal tells in these interviews that you've learned in this chapter.

Chapter 12 –
How to Use Boundaries to Protect Yourself from Predators

By Chuck O'Neill

"There are boundaries to the individual soul. And in our dealings with each other we generally respect these boundaries. It is characteristic of—and prerequisite for—mental health both that our own ego boundaries should be clear and that we should clearly recognize the boundaries of others. We must know where we end and others begin."
— M. Scott Peck, People of the Lie

"Boundaries are to protect life, not to limit pleasures."
— Edwin Louis Cole

He seemed like a nice guy at first.

At least that was what Cynthia thought when she met Bob outside the restaurant for their first date. He'd held the door for her and even pulled out her chair. Very chivalrous.

He was handsome, too, with baby blue eyes and soft dirty-blonde hair that looked slightly messy, like he'd just finished a pickup football game with friends. Plus, he actually looked like his online profile. Cynthia smiled. So far, two thumbs up.

Then the tide began to turn.

When the waiter came, Bob ordered for the two of them even though Cynthia laughed and said she should probably order for herself since she was picky about food.

Bob shook his head vehemently. "No—I insist. I know this restaurant pretty well. I know what's good and what's not. Trust me."

They'd just met; how could he possibly know what she liked? Cynthia shrugged it off. He was probably just trying to impress her.

While they waited for their food, they covered the standard first-date topics: jobs, hobbies, favorite vacation spots, favorite movies, etc.

Then, just as Cynthia started to relax, Bob winked and asked, "So would you say you're a sexually adventurous person?"

"Um," Cynthia shifted in her seat. "I'm not sure I'm comfortable talking about that on a first date."

Bob laughed, "Oh, come on, I'm just having some fun. No harm meant." He held up his hands in mock horror. "I didn't realize you were such a prude."

Cynthia rushed to defend herself. "I'm not a prude—I just don't know you yet. So that topic is a little personal."

Bob leaned in and placed a hand on her knee under the table. "Okay, so you're not a prude—good to know."

Before Cynthia could process what that meant, their meals arrived. Bob had ordered the almond-encrusted salmon for both of them—and Cynthia had to admit that it was excellent. However, she nearly dropped her fork when Bob leaned over and helped himself to her fingerling potatoes.

"Do you mind?" he asked with that boyish grin. "I know a tiny thing like you probably can't eat carbs and stay so thin."

What could she say? What woman didn't like to be called 'tiny' or 'thin'?

Bob did seem genuinely interested in her and plied her with questions throughout the meal. So much so that by the end of the meal, Bob knew everything from where Cynthia worked to how she liked her coffee to which dog park she visited on the weekends. However, when Cynthia tried to ask Bob some questions about himself, she was left with one- or two-word answers.

Cynthia knew practically nothing about Bob.

"Shall we go then?" he asked as he downed the last of his wine. "I know a great little coffee shop down the road. It's pretty quiet this time of night, so we'll probably have the whole place to ourselves."

Cynthia hesitated, not entirely sure she wanted to continue the date. Bob was coming on a bit too strong for her taste.

"Thanks, but I think I'm done for the night. It was a lovely dinner—thank you." She rose.

He looked crestfallen.

"Come on now. If I'm going to spring for a five-star dinner, the least you can do is humor me with a late-night coffee. I'm really enjoying getting to know you."

"Well ...." she wavered. Bob was right; he had spent a fortune on this dinner. And all he was trying to do was to get to know her better. What was the harm, really?

"All right," she gave in.

They rose and Bob helped her put her coat on, leaning just a bit too close for Cynthia's comfort. Maybe it was the wine talking already, she thought. He was certainly forceful.

The two had agreed to meet at the restaurant (even though Bob had originally offered to pick Cynthia up at her home). So Cynthia started off towards her car.

"Should I follow you then?" she asked, fumbling to get her keys out of her purse. Bob's hand came down over the purse.

"What? What kind of date would I be if I let you drive yourself? The place is just up the street. Come on—hop in my car. I'll drop you off back here when we're done." He winked at her. "Provided, of course, you want to let me go tonight."

Cynthia felt trapped. If the coffee shop was just up the street, it would seem silly to take two separate cars. She would feel like an idiot getting into an argument over this, especially when Bob was clearly trying so hard to be charming.

Still, she hesitated. Seeing her uncertainty, Bob stepped in, put his arm around her and steered her away from her car towards his.

"Come on now. Don't make me beg. Honestly, I'm a good guy. I'll be on my best behavior—I promise."

Cynthia gave in and let him guide her to his car. It turned out to be the biggest mistake she ever made. Bob turned out to be a sexual predator who assaulted her that night after driving them—not to the coffee shop—but to the dead-end road where he'd planned to go after he'd gotten her in his car.

What Are Boundaries?

Many times when I talk about boundaries in my seminars or classes, people aren't exactly sure what I mean. We live in a world that has very murky boundaries, and not a lot of people talk about them. However, that doesn't mean they don't exist.

Boundaries are very real. They can be used to protect you and guard your emotional, physical, and mental well-being.

What exactly are boundaries?

A boundary is something that protects you—it keeps the bad out and lets the good in.

For example, your skin is a physical boundary for your organs, brain, and heart. If you have a fence around your yard, that is a physical boundary for your property. It protects your lawn from the dog next door leaving you a nice little brown present.

Your personal space is a boundary.

For example, how many times have you met someone (like an annoying sales agent or a socially inept party guest) who stood unusually close to you—so close you felt the overwhelming urge to step back and farther away from them?

That was an example of your personal-space boundary being violated.

Boundaries can vary depending on our relationships with different people.

For example, your spouse or lover can usually stand much closer to you than a perfect stranger can. And chances are you will let your family or close friends say things to you that you'd never let a stranger say.

There are four different types of boundaries:

#1: Physical Boundaries: These can include your personal space, your physical body, or anything around you (e.g., your car, your house, a stall in a washroom, a dressing room, your clothes, etc.).

#2: Mental Boundaries: These boundaries are your beliefs, your personal philosophy, the way you think, how you view yourself and life around you, what you want from life, etc.

It can also include the proper mental balance that's right for you. For example, if you've done something mentally taxing for a certain time, you may need to do something 'mindless' for a while to restore your personal mental balance.

#3: Emotional Boundaries: These are similar to mental boundaries, but they concern your emotional balance. For example, when someone is using guilt, obligation, or fear to manipulate you into doing something you don't want to do (as Bob was doing in the example above), they are crossing an emotional boundary.

When someone expects you to make them happy instead of taking responsibility for their own emotional health, it's an example of crossing emotional boundaries.

#4: Social/Religious Boundaries: These have to do with different cultures. For example, in certain countries, women have a boundary that requires them to keep certain parts of their bodies covered.

If you are a woman and you go into one of these countries and don't cover up in this way, you are violating that country's religious and cultural boundary, and it may not go well for you.

As another example, in some cultures it's considered a major boundary violation for a woman to touch a man (with a hug or handshake, for example) who is not her husband.

You must always keep these types of boundaries in mind when dealing with other people in different countries, cultures, and religions.

How Do Boundaries Protect You?

First of all, you have to be aware of your own boundaries. You have to know who you are, what you want, what you deem appropriate behavior, etc. Never be afraid to work out your own boundaries, even if other people have different ones than you do.

You are an individual, and you have every right to have your own boundaries for your life. But you have to know what they are before you can communicate them to someone else.

In our example above, Cynthia had a boundary: She didn't want a total stranger coming to her house for the first date. She didn't feel comfortable with that, and she smartly enforced it with Bob.

However, she then violated her boundary about not getting into a car with a complete stranger on the first night they met, and she paid a price for it. Because she had already let him violate certain boundaries, Bob didn't think twice about going further and trying to violate her sexual boundaries later on.

Another example of knowing your physical boundaries is keeping to the five-foot rule. This rule states you should always keep five to six feet between yourself and a stranger who approaches you on the street or in a deserted area if at all possible.

Why?

Because if the guy (or girl) is simply asking a harmless question, like what time it is, they shouldn't need to get that close to you. And if they are trying to get that close to you, it's for a reason—most likely because they want to grab you, hit you, push you, or otherwise attack you. And they can't do it from five feet away.

So knowing your own boundaries—physical, emotional, or mental—is step number one in using them to protect yourself.

The second step is communicating these boundaries to others—sometimes very clearly if the situation calls for it.

For example, Cynthia did communicate her discomfort with Bob's sexual comment at the beginning of their date by telling him she wasn't comfortable with that topic. However, she should have not ignored the fact that he didn't respect her boundary (by touching her knee and calling her a prude). If someone is continually ignoring your boundaries, especially if you've made them clear, that is a warning signal.

How Do You Communicate Your Boundaries?

You may communicate your boundaries in several ways. You can state them out loud for people.

For example, if you aren't comfortable meeting a client at his home, you can tell him when scheduling an appointment that you never meet clients in their homes. Blame company policy if you have to, but make sure he knows that you will not meet him in his home—ever.

Or let's say you're getting out of your car in a parking lot one day and you notice a stranger approaching you. You decide to use the 'five-foot rule' boundary we talked about above.

To state that boundary, you may want to ask the stranger to stay where they are or ask them to stay five feet away from you. You might look silly, but you'll be clearly stating your boundary, which is a huge turn-off for predators looking for a victim.

You can state your boundaries physically, for example, by putting space between you and another person, like a physical object. They would then have to move around the object to get to you.

The Importance of Enforcing Your Boundaries

Once you've clearly stated your boundaries, it's important to enforce your boundaries, especially if the person is not listening to you and respecting your boundaries. None of us likes to do this. However, it is essential and could protect you from something much worse down the road.

There are many ways to enforce your boundaries, but it has nothing to do with controlling the other person or forcing them to do something. Enforcing your boundaries is all about what you can do.

Here are some examples of how you might decide to enforce your boundaries:

- ◊ Remove yourself from the situation.
- ◊ Set a time limit on how long you'll talk to a certain person.
- ◊ Leave the room.
- ◊ Fill out a police report.
- ◊ Don't pick up the phone when it rings.
- ◊ Ask another person to stay with you during a meeting.
- ◊ Stop cleaning up the other person's mess and let them experience the consequences of their own actions.
- ◊ Don't pay for somebody else's stuff.
- ◊ Change the locks.
- ◊ Change your phone number.
- ◊ Stick to certain 'safe' subjects when in conversation with a certain person.
- ◊ Refuse to listen when somebody wants to dump all of their emotional baggage on you.

Enforcing your boundaries may seem tough, and it may actually take some work and cost something on your part. However, it is your responsibility.

I'll give you an example of enforcing a physical boundary. Kate and I once moved to a home that didn't have a backyard fence. Practically every night that summer (much to our surprise) the neighbourhood kids would go running through our yard.

They would play hide and seek around our house—even jump off our deck—screaming so loudly we'd come running to see if they'd hurt themselves. (If they had by the way, we would have been legally liable because they were on our property.)

We asked them to stop several times. However, kids being kids, after a few weeks they'd be back at it, screaming like ban-

shoes as they raced across our deck on a new adventure. This went on for months. Finally, after my wife's best friend screamed from the kitchen one night after catching a boy looking in at her through the patio door, we decided it was time to enforce our boundaries.

So we put up a fence. The result? No more neighbourhood kids running through our yard anymore. That was an example of protecting what was ours by enacting a physical boundary. It was expensive and a bit of a pain, but it was our responsibility.

Another example of boundary enforcement is emotional, not allowing others to use you, holding them accountable for their actions, and refusing to clean up their messes for them.

For example, let's say you have a coworker who can't seem to pull her own weight at the office. She asks you for one quick favor on a group project, and before you know it, you're regularly finishing up her work for her so that she doesn't get in trouble and the project gets done.

This may be okay for the first few times. The problem is that you're now doing your job and half of hers as well. And all the time you're spending at work is making you grouchy, tired, and depressed.

That coworker is violating your boundaries in this situation. But it's up to you to enforce them. You can't blame her for violating your boundaries if you aren't ready to enforce them.

In this situation, you enforce your boundary by telling her that you can no longer do her work for her. Then you let her live with the consequences. She may try to make you feel guilty. She may threaten that projects won't get finished. But you still have to stand your ground and not allow your emotional boundaries to get trampled on.

Maybe she'll lose her job. Maybe she'll find someone else to do her work for her. Maybe she'll even get her butt in gear and do the work herself. Who knows? That's not your responsibility. Your responsibility is to enforce your own boundaries.

So to summarize, when it comes to boundaries, you have three tasks:

#1: Know your boundaries.

#2: Clearly state your boundaries to others, making sure they understand them.

#3: Enforce your boundaries by doing what you can do.

How Can You Use Boundaries to Protect Yourself?

Almost every attack is preceded by one, if not several, boundary violations, whether physical, emotional, mental, or social. Boundary violations—especially when it comes to predators—are all about control. They want it. If you let them take it, they will take more and more until sometimes, it's too late.

Cynthia's story is a powerful example of someone who ignored the violation of her boundaries to her own peril.

(Please note that I'm not saying in any way that she deserved to be attacked. In fact, Bob was a very skillful manipulator. However, this is a great example of how predators will lead up to an attack by crossing boundaries.)

While not every 'Bob' is a predator, the one in this case turned out to be a particularly nasty one—a sexual sociopath who had tested Cynthia's boundaries from the first moment they'd met. Cynthia had actually done pretty well at first—not letting Bob pick her up, not giving him her address. She even called him on his inappropriate sexual comment.

However, she failed to notice Bob's continual boundary violations all night:

- ◊ He insisted on ordering for her and ignored her protest that she wanted to order for herself.

- ◊ He made a highly inappropriate sexual comment and then laughed off her protest about it.

- ◊ He then insulted her by calling her a prude, basically disrespecting the sexual boundary she had clearly laid out for him.

- ◊ He crossed her physical boundaries several times, including putting his hand on her knee not 10 minutes after they'd first met.

- ◊ He also closed his hand over her purse and wouldn't let her get her keys out. He put his arm around her and physically steered her towards his car.

- ◊ He also crossed her physical boundary by 'claiming' her food and eating from her plate (an act that would be fine if they'd been dating for several months—but highly inappropriate on a first date).

- ◊ He crossed her emotional boundary by making her feel obligated to go to the coffee shop with him (by reminding her he'd paid for an expensive dinner, making her feel that she owed him).

- ◊ He did not respect her desire to drive in separate cars.

- ◊ And he made her feel like she would be making a big deal over nothing ("It's just down the street") if she wanted to go in separate cars (minimizing her feelings).

Bob was a major boundary violator that night, giving off several warning signals which Cynthia could have picked up on—if she'd known what to look for.

Now, not every guy who does these things is a predator; he might just be an arrogant jackass. But if someone is continually disrespecting your boundaries, take it as a red flag and consider taking action to remove yourself from the situation.

If you can't remove yourself from the situation, you may decide to set up your own, more stringent boundaries that will protect you.

For example, if there is someone who emotionally and mentally taxes you every time you're together, but you have to see them, you may want to enforce time boundaries:

"I'll see them for only two hours once a month." Or "I'll speak with them only on the phone for 20 minutes, and then I'll make an excuse and get off the phone."

Or you may lay down boundaries like "I'll keep conversation to neutral topics like the weather and current events."

I once did a talk which included how to spot unhealthy people, sociopaths, and psychopaths in your life. I received feedback about a week later from a guy I'll call 'Mike'.

Mike admitted that from that talk, he'd suddenly realized that a friend of his was an unhealthy person—constantly lying, criticizing other people, and stirring up trouble just for the entertainment of watching the drama unfold.

Mike told me, "I'd never realized just how many problems my friend was causing, not just in his life, but mine as well. I suddenly realized that every time we hung out, I ended up feeling down about myself and just really crappy afterwards.

"He was affecting me really badly. I've since put up a boundary that I'll hang out with him only once a month. I've already noticed a huge shift in my life—the world doesn't look so hopeless."

Remember, boundaries are for your protection, and it's your right to set them in order to protect yourself.

So now that you know about the skills of Awareness and Boundaries and Body Language, what happens when, for some reason, these fail and you get to the 'C' stage—Confrontation?

That's coming up in the next chapter. You're going to learn verbal and visual skills to help you de-escalate a confrontation situation before it turns violent.

Important Points:

- ◊ Boundaries are there to protect you; they let the good in and keep the bad out.

- ◊ You can have physical, mental, emotional, and religious or cultural boundaries.

- ◊ It's up to you to know your boundaries and to make sure that others know about them too.

- ◊ It's up to you to respect other people's boundaries while recognizing your own.

- ◊ It's up to you to clearly state your boundaries and then take steps to enforce them if they are not respected.

- ◊ Most attacks are preceded by several blatant boundary violations.

- ◊ Predators will purposely violate your boundaries (emotional, physical, mental, or social) to see how you react. If you let them violate your boundaries, they will go further until sometimes it's too late and you are harmed.

- ◊ If someone continually violates or disrespects your boundaries, this is a red flag. You should remove yourself from the situation or the person. If that is not possible, you should enforce more stringent boundaries (like limiting your time with them) in order to protect yourself.

Boundaries Exercise:

Take some time to think about—or write down—your personal boundaries. Here are some questions to guide you:

#1: What are my physical boundaries?

#2: What are my emotional boundaries?

#3: What are my mental boundaries?

#4: What are my cultural/religious boundaries?

#5: Are there any areas of my life where someone is currently violating my boundaries?

#6: What can I do to enforce my boundaries?

#7: What are some past instances where someone has violated my boundaries? What did I do about it?

#8: Am I currently violating anyone else's boundaries?

Chapter 13 –
Confrontation – Using Visual and Verbal Skills to Avoid an Attack

By Chuck O'Neill

<u>Fact</u>: *According to The Little Black Book of Violence by Lawrence A. Kane and Kris Wilder, men are more likely to be victimized by a stranger, whereas women are more likely to be victimized by a friend, acquaintance, or intimate.*

"If you walk upright with larger movements, swinging your arms and legs and having your front open, you will project that you could defend yourself if necessary and so are less likely to be attacked."
— Allan and Barbara Pease, *The Definitive Book of Body Language*

So what happens when, for whatever reason, the 'A' and 'B' skills don't work and you get to the 'C'—Confrontation?

The good news is that you still have options. You can still avoid a physical attack.

The first option we'll talk about is using verbal and visual skills to confront.

Remember Cheryl, the real estate agent from chapter six? While she didn't necessarily get to the ultimate confrontation with her open-house straggler, she did use verbal and visual skills to fail her interview and send the predator on his way.

For example, she faced him head on and looked him straight in the eye when speaking to him. She made sure she never turned her back on him.

She used a strong, confident tone. She asked him questions, effectively putting him on the spot and forcing him to go on the defensive instead of the offensive. Her questions tripped him up as he was intent on maneuvering her into a certain position. By forcing him to answer her questions, she was effectively throwing him off his game. He couldn't be in both attack and defense mode.

Then there was Kyle from chapter six, who also failed his predator interview by standing up to the bar bully. By visually positioning himself into a proper fight stance, he showed he was ready to fight should the guy come at him.

He also stood tall and tried to take up as much space as possible. He used his verbal skills to challenge his attacker and show that he was confident he would win in a fight (after trying to talk him down to no avail).

So how can you use verbal and visual skills to avoid an attack?

As with any situation, there is no one right formula—do this and he'll always do that, say this and he'll always say that. You have to use your awareness skills and instincts in every situation.

However, facing the person head on is not only a powerful signal to them that you'll be trouble if they attack, it also helps you better see the situation should an attack happen (including possible exits, improvised weapons, etc.).

Verbally, a strong, confident tone also signals you'll be trouble because you're not afraid to back down. Keeping them on the verbal defensive (if possible) by asking them questions can buy you time to plan an escape. It also psychologically forces them into a defensive position versus an offensive position (for attack).

A part of the visual skills you can use at this stage has to do with how you appear to the predator. You can use subtle body language cues to de-escalate a tense situation. They include:

#1: Keeping Your Hands in the Belly Button or Navel Plane: This is actually a technique used by experienced speakers and politicians to make them appear more trustworthy and believable to their audiences.

When you're trying to talk a person down, keep your hands moving in what I call the navel plane of space. This is the area extending out from your belly button (or just below) in front of you and to the sides. There are several reasons for this.

First of all, this makes you look calmer and more trustworthy to the other person. As humans we have a tendency to mirror what we see others do. So if someone sees you acting calm (versus gesturing wildly up higher in the chest or shoulder area), they are more likely to feel some of their own energy dissipate.

Secondly, it affects your vocal tone, keeping it calmer and more reassuring. According to body language expert Mark Bowden in his book *Winning Body Language*, when we keep our hands and gestures located within this plane:

"Because of the interconnected nature of the physical system, your vocal tone is affected congruently with the Gesture-Plane [navel plane]. Therefore, your whole vocal tone becomes more calming and trustworthy."

Lastly, keeping your hands in this plane, because of the same mechanisms that affect vocal tone, can help keep *you* feeling stable and calm, counteracting the stress that you will no doubt be feeling in a tense situation.

#2: Keep Your Hands Open and Up—Showing Your Palms: This is also another way to show trustworthiness. The palms-up-and-open gesture has been used for years and dates back to when warriors would display their open palms as a way to show they were not holding their weapons.

Basically, it says to the other person, "I'm not trying to hurt you. I want no trouble." This can also help to diffuse a situation.

#3: The Subtle Nodding Effect: People like people who agree with them. They also like people who listen to them (because so many people don't listen these days!).

If someone is complaining to you or venting, a subtle nod on your part can make them feel validated and help calm them down. It also unconsciously makes them feel that you're on their side because you're agreeing with them. So they may go from seeing you as the adversary to part of their team.

Basically, when you nod in agreement with someone, it fosters positive feelings on their part towards you, which can also help deflate a tense situation.

However, you have to be careful here and only nod if the situation calls for it.

For example, if someone is attacking you verbally and threatening you personally, it may not be the right time to nod and stoke the fire by agreeing with them.

However, if they're venting about the company, the bar, their girlfriend, or something else that isn't related to you, nodding calmly may be a great way to help diffuse their energy and make them feel heard.

You also have to keep the nods subtle as nodding energetically may only increase their energy. But a subtle, occasional nod can go a long way towards calming someone down. It may also buy you time to assess the situation more accurately.

So those are some of the more subtle visual and body language skills you can use to diffuse a tense situation. Before we get into a few more things you can do, let's break down the different types of dynamics happening in confrontation situations:

#1: Male vs. Male – The Alpha-Dog Effect: A male vs. male confrontation is usually very different from a female vs. male confrontation (or even female vs. female). When two men are confronting each other, you have a situation that I call 'the alpha-dog effect'.

Most men feel a tremendous pressure to be the 'alpha', or top dog. We grow up with it. We compete for it. Being the top dog (the richest, the buffest, the smartest, the strongest) is ultimate success for us.

Being second to the top dog doesn't count. There is no second best.

And if you put that alpha-dog drive into an insecure guy and add a hefty dose of alcohol or adrenaline, he may end up pummeling you into the ground and happily going to jail, just to prove that he was the alpha.

Too many times a verbal confrontation is escalated into a physical altercation between men because of this alpha-dog effect—even if neither one of them wants it. Insults start flying and egos get involved until one party is effectively backed into a corner. He then feels he has no choice but to escalate to physical violence to defend his honor, even if he doesn't want to. That's how strong the male alpha drive is.

So what can you do? There are several surefire ways you can de-escalate this alpha-dog scenario and prevent it from getting to the physical level.

First of all, use the above two tips: Keep your hands gesturing in the belly-button plane with palms open and up.

Secondly, avoid any territorial displays like leaning against the frame of a door or putting your foot on his chair leg (or the chair leg at his table). Leaning against any object that belongs to someone else can be perceived as dominating and intimidating.

I'm not saying you have to be a pansy here, guys. But you have to realize that taking an insult to your ego may just be better than spending the night in the hospital (or even in jail).

Try to back off, and if you think the guy is just an arrogant ass, concede him the point. Tell him you don't want trouble and see what he does. Nine times out of 10 he will back off (especially if he's just an everyday dumbass attacker we talked about before). He doesn't want a fight; he just wants to look like 'the man' in front of his buddies.

There are occasions, however, where he won't back down, even if you're showing your palms-up submissive body language and avoiding territorial displays.

This guy may be one of the few that takes submission on your part as a challenge to push further. These guys are bullies and will back down only if they think you're willing and ready to stand your ground.

Go back to our example of Kyle, who faced down the belligerent, drunk muscleman who'd shoved his girlfriend in the bar. Kyle tried the first approach, telling the guy they didn't want trouble (verbal).

That didn't work because this particular bully took submission as an invitation to dish out more abuse. Kyle knew his only option was to bully the guy back and use visual, physical, and verbal skills to try and make him back down. So he stood up, assumed the martial arts defensive pose (effectively demonstrating he was indeed ready for a confrontation), and verbally insulted the bully.

This had the effect of making Kyle look like he was confident and skilled, planting doubt in the muscleman's head that perhaps Kyle would cause some serious damage in a fight.

It also had the effect of forcing the bully to make the first move.

Just remember if you choose to confront (or demonstrate physical confrontation like Kyle did), you also have to be ready to back up your actions with physical skills. We don't always get a bully to back down as Kyle did. That's why I tell people this is your last option after trying to talk them down and displaying submissive non-confrontational body language.

Force Them to Make the First Move

This is a very important psychological attack tool. When you show that you're ready for a fight—but you aren't going to make the first move—it forces the predator to consider the consequences of his actions if he initiates the fight.

While I am not legal counsel, keep in mind that in general:

In a physical fight, the one who attacks first is often the one who is legally liable.

Also consider that any unwanted touch could be considered a form of assault.

The one who attacks first is usually the one who gets charged and goes to jail. The one who is simply defending himself for all to see is usually in the clear. And if your predator has had any physical altercations before, he's going to know this.

You generally don't want to 'egg' or coax your opponent on. If you do, this may be seen as aggravating the situation. However, you do want to make sure your attacker knows that he is the one who will be making the first move.

By forcing a guy to make the first move, you can often make them think twice as they don't want to be held accountable for their actions.

I used this strategy when doing a security job for UFC fighter Chuck Liddell a few years back. Mr. Liddell was signing autographs for a large crowd of people who had been waiting in line for hours.

Because of time constraints, we had to, unfortunately,

change gears midway during the day and tell people they could have only two items signed instead of four or five. We wanted to make sure everyone got through the line as Mr. Liddell had to leave in a couple of hours.

One young guy in the line didn't like this change of plans and started to cause problems, complaining loudly and trying to stir things up. I immediately took him aside, knowing that he was quickly becoming agitated and the situation could get physical.

By removing him from the crowd, I ensured that he wouldn't stir up more discontent with his words and negative energy. I also dulled the alpha-dog drive from him. (Because his buddies were not in earshot, he wouldn't be forced into provoking a fight with me just to prove that he was a tough guy in front of them.)

Then I forced him to make the first move.

"Sir, I understand you're upset," I said. "But unfortunately those are the rules—two signed items only. We don't have time for more."

"That f***ing sucks. I've been waiting over two hours. I'm gonna get whatever I want signed, and you can't stop me."

"No," I said, "you're not. Two items only."

He looked me over and issued the challenge. "I'll do what I want, man. What are you gonna do about it?"

I looked him directly in the eye and firmly, calmly asked, "Are you asking me to remove you from the premises, sir?"

He faltered a bit, but the bravado held up.

"You wouldn't dare ..."

"Are you asking me to remove you from the premises, sir?"

Keeping my voice calm and non-confrontational, I began to move my body slowly into position.

"You can't. You wouldn't." But he was quickly losing steam as he noticed the change in my body language.

I had moved into position and was fully ready at that moment to take him down physically and remove him from the premises. However, I was going to make sure that he would be the one attacking so that he would be the one responsible for me removing him from the premises.

It also hadn't escaped his notice that I had asked the question loudly enough for others to hear. So now there were witnesses watching to verify that he had instigated a physical fight with me.

I asked a third time.

"Are you saying that you want me to physically remove you from the premises, sir?"

I watched as his shoulders suddenly gave way and the manic energy drained from his face. I knew we'd just averted a physical altercation.

He shook his head and mumbled, "No."

"Very good, sir, I appreciate that. I would hate for you to spend all this time waiting for Mr. Liddell and then not get what you came for. I know it's frustrating, and I know you've been waiting a long time. So I'm going to personally escort you to Mr. Liddell now so you won't have to wait any longer."

He perked up with that news. I allowed him to save face by telling him I knew he'd waited a long time already. By escorting him personally to Mr. Liddell, his bruised ego was mended somewhat. I didn't do this to reward his bad behavior. He'd already proven he was a potential problem. As Mr. Liddell's security detail, I wasn't about to let him go near my client without ensuring that I was in between them, heading off any potential problems.

It was also my way of alerting my client to a potential problem. Mr. Liddell knew the signal—that if I escorted someone personally to him, that person was considered a possible danger. This alerted my client to be extra careful and spend as little time as possible with this man.

The man may have thought he was saving a few minutes of time, but he actually lost out as Mr. Liddell gave him the bare minimum of his time and did not take a picture with him.

So by using the verbal strategy of forcing this man to instigate the attack, I was able to de-escalate the situation. We averted a potential physical scuffle, and the man got to save face in front of his friends. It was a win-win.

Remind Them of the Consequences

An additional tool you can use in these kinds of situations is reminding your potential attacker of the consequences of their actions. You may want to say something like:

"Do you want me to defend myself if you attack me? Everyone here will know you started it, which is what they'll tell the police."

Or:

"Do you really want to get charged with assault? Because if you attack me, that's what will happen. Am I really worth that much to you?"

Notice in these statements I used the word 'attack' instead of 'fight'. Most guys are up for a fight.

But when you use the word 'attack', you're subtly changing the situation, implying that he is the attacker and you're just the defender. Most guys don't have a problem thinking of themselves as fighters, but they don't want to think of themselves as attackers.

You might also say something like, "Look man, neither of us wants all the trouble this is going to cause, so let's just forget about it, okay?" You're subtly reminding him of the consequences of his actions if he attacks.

You could also be blunter with something like this, "Look man, there are cameras everywhere in this place recording everything. That could mean a lawsuit or jail time for us both, so let's just forget it, okay?"

By reminding him that he's on camera, you're again subtly reminding him of the consequences of his actions, should he come after you.

Another thing you can do is show respect. Every guy wants to be respected. Unfortunately, however, it's in short supply these days. If you show respect and talk to him like he's a buddy and like you're both on the same page, you're much more likely to talk him down.

So what do you do if using these methods (letting him have the alpha-dog position, forcing him to make the first move, reminding him of the consequences, and showing respect) doesn't work?

Then chances are high that your attacker is not an everyday dumbass. He's more likely a sociopath, a criminal, or a physically driven attacker. So you may have to stand up to him and show him you're willing to give it right back to him in order to get him to back down.

However, again, this is a last resort as facing up to someone in this way can be very confrontational and, in fact, escalate things. Use this only when you've tried the other methods above.

This is the one thing that worked for Kyle in the example above because his attacker interpreted his submission as an invitation to keep going. So the important thing is to be on red alert, watching for what kind of predator you're facing and testing out what works and what doesn't.

#2: Male vs. Female – It's All about Control

Things are very different if you get into a male vs. female (or even female vs. female) confrontation. You don't have the alpha-dog effect. But you do have the issue of control. In most situations where a man attacks a woman, it's about control. He wants to control her—her boundaries, her body, her behavior, her wallet, her emotions, etc.

If you understand this, it can help you understand when to back down and when to stand up to him.

Many predators will try to take control of small things first before escalating the situation and taking control of you at the next level. If you cut them off at the small things, you can often stop them from escalating and taking control of larger things.

For example, in the last chapter when Cynthia went out with Bob, he was trying to control her from the very start.

He wanted to order for her, pick her up at her house, eat off her plate, etc. He ignored her sexual boundaries with his talk and his touch (asserting his control in that area as well). And for the most part, she let him—which was a signal to Bob that he could keep going.

Now contrast that with our real estate agent, Cheryl. She did let her open-house straggler in at the last minute, which did give him some control of the situation. But once he was in, she quickly recovered and controlled the situation. She didn't back down. She didn't turn her back on him. And she let him know that he'd soon be facing another man—her husband—if he stuck around.

By controlling the situation, she managed to turn her predator off and send him on his way, before things escalated into an attack.

This is also a great example of how you can turn things around, even if you make some initial mistakes.

So what if you do get into a confrontation? What are some other verbal and visual tools you can use to de-escalate the situation?

Here are a few things you can try, keeping in mind that the situation dictates which ones you choose to use:

◊ Maintain steady, calm eye contact with the potential attacker.

◊ Ask them questions to determine what they really want. Show respect for what they're saying—it may deflate them to realize that someone is actually listening to them.

◊ Keep your voice tone calm and low (which helps you sound authoritative, especially for women who tend to have higher-pitched voices than men). It may also help to keep your arms moving in the navel plane, which again makes you seem more authoritative and calm than if you're moving them in the chest or head plane.

◊ Phrase things in the attacker's best interest. For example, "I know you're upset, but do you want to spend the rest of your life paying for this?" or "This isn't worth the trouble, especially for someone of your skills."

◊ Ask questions to throw them off. For example, if they're making lewd comments to you, try asking them something completely out of the blue like, "What do you think about the state of affairs in Iran?" It interrupts their thought process, forces them to slow down and process, and may give you a few extra seconds to get away.

◊ Display territorial body language. Unlike the male vs. male situation, if you're a woman feeling like a man is trying to bully you, it might make sense to start displaying territorial body language: feet wide apart, arms crossed, leaning against or over your table. By showing strong territorial body language, you are telling him that he won't easily be able to dominate you.

◊ If all else fails, make sure they know that you're going to be a lot of trouble should they decide to attack (standing tall, taking up physical space, looking them directly in the eye, etc.).

Are there situations where you should back down and give in verbally to a predator? Yes.

And as you should know by now, there is no set formula that works for every situation, every time. Each situation is different, even though there are general principles you can use to help yourself.

Sometimes it's better to tell a predator what they want to hear and not challenge them, just to keep them calm while you observe them, look for weaknesses, and make plans to get away.

Just understand two things: First of all, it's usually about him wanting to control you. Don't give him control unless you're using it as a stall tactic to get out of the situation later on.

Secondly, remember that he isn't thinking like you, so don't expect him to conform to the polite rules of society that you conform to. (For example, he won't be honest, nice or polite. He will almost certainly lie to you.)

Female vs. female physical attacks are not as common as the above two situations. Most female vs. female attacks are on the psychological and emotional attack level (like our situation with Kelly stealing Jenna's bank job and reputation in chapter seven). It can be about control here also, but it can also be about taking something from you that they want.

In these types of situations, the 'confrontation' is rarely physical. So the best way to defend yourself is to spot an envious, dangerous, sociopathic, or narcissistic person ahead of time before they have the chance to worm their way into your life and destroy it. Then get away as soon as you can.

What's Driving Them?

When looking to de-escalate any confrontation situation, whether it's male vs. male, female vs. male, or female vs. female, one thing you'll want to discover, if the situation permits, is this:

What's driving them?

This isn't just so that you can talk them down and give them what they want. It's also so that you know what you're dealing with so that you can make a better call on what your action should be.

For example, do they simply want your wallet? Do they want to appear like the alpha dog in front of their friends? Or is the driving force more complex? For example, maybe they want to exert control over you and get you to do what they want.

Are they driven by a physical addiction like drugs? Then how determined do you think they'll be going up against someone who just wants to look good in front of their friends?

Are they driven specifically because it's you (e.g., they're jealous, they want your job or your boyfriend, etc.)?

Or are they driven just to take and you happened to be the first person they came across? In that case, they will be more easily persuaded to move on to another victim because one victim is just as good as another.

You can't always know exactly what is driving someone. But if possible, try to discover this information because you'll then have a better idea of what you're up against when trying to talk them down.

So what happens when you hit the bottom of the barrel, when the crap hits the fan and things get physical? You're going to learn how you can handle that in the next chapter.

Important Points:

◊ Even if an altercation gets to the confrontation point, there are still things you can do (verbal and physical) in order to de-escalate the situation and avoid a physical attack.

◊ Subtle body language, like the navel-plane gesture, or palms up and nodding, can often de-escalate a tense situation.

◊ There are often different underlying factors in a male vs. male confrontation (the alpha-dog effect), a male vs. female (the issue of control), or female vs. female confrontation.

◊ Always force a potential predator to make the first move. They will then be forced to consider if they really want to attack you, and you will be better off legally if an attack does occur.

◊ There are certain situations where you may want to back down or submit to an attacker to see how he reacts or to give yourself time to get away.

◊ In the case of emotional or psychological attacks, there may not be a confrontation; you have to try and spot these kinds of predators early in the game and get yourself away from them.

◊ Always trust your gut instinct in any attack situation, and don't expect your predator to think like you would.

◊ Try to figure out your attacker's intentions when devising a plan to get away from the situation.

Exercise Your Confrontation Skills (Covertly)

For the next few days try using the body language skills you learned in this chapter when you interact with different people.

Keep your gestures in the navel plane when speaking to office colleagues, friends, the difficult receptionist at the dental office, etc. Use the open-palm and palm-up gestures and see how people react to you. Nod subtly when you're asking them to do something they might not want to do for you.

Notice how people react to you. Are they calmer? Friendlier? Easier to get along with?

One caveat: use your skills for good here, not for evil. I'm not advocating you go around trying to manipulate people! I just want you to start learning how you can contribute to the energy of a situation and even bring that energy down should things turn hostile.

Chapter 14 –
Physical Confrontations –
What to Do When All Else Fails

By Chuck O'Neill

"Extraordinary people survive under the most terrible circumstances and they become more extraordinary because of it."
— Robertson Davies

So what happens if you get down to the last 'C' and the Confrontation goes physical? What happens if the attack occurs and you find yourself a victim of a vicious predator?

There are still some things you can do. You still have control. This chapter is going to help give you options so that if it ever does come down to a confrontation, you can make the best decision for your situation.

First of all, this chapter is not going to cover physical self-defense moves. We're going to cover psychological self-defense strategies here, strategies with the ultimate goal of keeping you alive.

If you want to know physical moves, I'd encourage you to take a regular martial arts class. (I'm partial to Wing Chun because it's so effective in a street fight.) Or learn some simple self-defense moves and practice them on a regular basis over and over again. That way it will be easier to perform them under a high-stress situation.

However, this chapter is all about teaching you some simple strategies to use when an attack happens to ensure you come out alive on the other end.

Here are some of my hard and fast 'survival rules' if you ever get into a physical confrontation:

#1: Don't *Ever* Let Yourself Be Taken to a Secondary Location: This is the worst thing you can do. Don't get in that car, no matter what he says. Don't go with him, even if he claims he'll let you go if you do. Don't use your keys to open your apartment door in front of him, even if he says he won't come in.

Nine times out of 10, a secondary location is where the most physical damage happens. It's where most victims are killed, raped, or beaten.

Why? Because a secondary location will be quiet and out of the way with no witnesses. You can bet on it.

When you're on the street, even if you're in a fringe area where there aren't a lot of people, an attacker still doesn't have total control of the location. People could still come along. There could still be a camera in a convenience store or a bank to catch him. This gives you some leverage in that situation because he's not in total control of the area.

If you go with him to a secondary location, you've just lost your leverage. You have nothing going for you, and he has absolutely no reason NOT to hurt you. In fact, he has more incentive to hurt you and possibly kill you in order to cover up what he's done.

#2: Once You Make the Decision to Fight Back, Go All the Way and Don't Stop Until Your Attacker Has Been Disabled

Here's a fact most people don't know:

When shot (or stabbed), most attackers will still keep coming at you for several seconds after they are hit. You *have* to finish the job.

If you're attacked and you decide this is the right moment to fight back, make the commitment and go all the way. Don't stop fighting until your attacker is on the ground and unable to come after you. You can't just knee a predator in the groin once and hope that will put him down. It might slow him down—it might even make him drop to the ground—but it won't stop him.

Why?

Because he's running on adrenaline, and adrenaline gives people super-endurance and super-strength.

Adrenaline is what gives an 80-year-old grandmother the strength to lift a car off her five-year-old grandchild. Adrenaline is what gives a boxer the strength to take more than 100 hits to the head and still keep fighting. Adrenaline is what gives soldiers the strength to keep advancing on the enemy when their bodies are riddled with shrapnel and bullet holes.

So while a knee to the groin might stop a predator in normal, everyday life, it won't stop him when his body is pumping with adrenaline.

This rule is particularly hard for women because it runs against their natures. I find this happens with many of the women I teach, in both martial arts and self-defense. They may fight back, but they never take it far enough.

They still have to fight their inborn training that says, "Be a nice girl" and "Hurting people is bad." That might be great for getting along in everyday life, but in an attack situation, all bets are off. Your survival is on the line, and you're going to have to fight like hell to save yourself.

Trust me, one tap to the groin of an adrenaline-driven, 250-pound man who's bent on raping you is not going to stop him. In fact, it might even enrage him. So if you decide fight, commit to it 100 percent.

Go all the way and don't stop fighting—with your legs, arms, voice, head, teeth, purse—whatever you have until your attacker stops and you have a chance to get away.

#3: Use a Distraction If You Can: If someone wants your wallet, throw it one way and then run another way. If someone is arguing with you, ask them a completely unrelated question. It will disrupt their thought process and force them to slow down, giving you time to get away.

I have a friend whose mother worked in Eaton's years ago. She told me the story of a botched robbery attempt one Christmas in her department.

Apparently, an older lady was working the ladies clothing register on her own. A young man in a black hoodie came in, flashed a knife, and ordered the woman to open the register and give him the money. For some reason, this woman reacted very differently than most people—including the robber—would expect.

She turned around and said, "Young man, WHERE is your mother? Does she know what you're up to tonight? You should be ashamed of yourself—get out of here before I call the police and they have to call your mother. Scoot now!"

The young robber was so thrown off by this feisty older woman's refusal to give him what he wanted that he just turned around and left, probably in shock.

Now this isn't something I recommend you try. But it's a great example of how throwing someone off by doing something completely unexpected can work in your favor.

#4: Have a Plan Ahead of Time: Once an attack occurs, you're already in the 'Black Zone'. Your adrenaline will be so high you won't be able to make a logical plan or think out a solid escape route. That's why it's so important to have a plan and go over it ahead of time.

For example, when I'm protecting a client, I research the area where we'll be days ahead of time. I know the terrain, the escape routes, the normal crowds, etc. I also have several plans of escape ahead of time, should we need to use them. In my mind, I rehearse every potential problem I can think of and map out what I'll do should any of these things happen.

You may not need to go into this much detail, but you can still have a plan ahead of time based on what you're facing. For example, if you work in a rough area of town, you might want to plan out strategies for what you'll do if you ever do get confronted with a mugger or attacker.

I know women who carry pepper spray or even aerosol hairspray in their hands when walking alone in rough parts of town. You may want to carry a 'fake' wallet to hand over to a mugger (with a few bills and old, expired credit cards).

You may want to have a group plan of what everyone in the family will do should something like a break-in occur (for example, a common meeting place, several exits the children can take, etc.).

My wife and I have code words we've agreed to use if either one of us is in danger. If she uses this code with me when I'm talking on the phone with her, I know to immediately hang up and call the police because she's in trouble.

When you have your plan, rehearse it in your mind continuously. Rehearsing the plan in your mind over and over again will help you know what to do if you ever do get attacked.

The bottom line is that if the worst happens, you won't be thinking straight. You will revert to your 'animal' limbic brain. So by rehearsing the plan ahead of time (even if only in your head), you're more likely to remember it when you need to.

"Victorious warriors win first and then go to war, while defeated warriors go to war first and then seek to win." — Sun Tzu, The Art of War

#5: Realize You *Do* Have Control: When people are attacked, they can very quickly feel helpless and victimized. They lose all sense of control. And when people lose control, hopelessness sets in, and then you have truly lost because you're unlikely to make any attempt to escape or defend yourself.

If you're attacked, it might not feel like it, but you do still have some form of control. You always have choices.

You have the choice to fight or submit. You have the choice to give up or try to escape. You have the choice to watch your attacker and try to find a weakness or to give up and wait for someone else to rescue you. You have the choice to go with them or say 'No'.

You still have a form of control. You still have many, many choices. And those choices can keep you alive.

Assert control in any way you can, even if it's just in some small way. Because that control will keep you moving forward instead of sinking into an abyss of despair. It will keep you thinking, trying to outsmart your attacker. When you feel like you have no control, hopelessness sets in and you give up. And then your attacker has already won.

Realize that your attacker has never truly won until you give up hope.

SAS Interrogation Training

I recently watched a documentary on the training that the British Special Air Service (SAS) go through when they are caught and interrogated by the enemy. One of the things they are taught is to always maintain some level of control.

This could be anything from defying the interrogator behind his back by sticking your tongue out at him, giving him the finger, covertly knocking things off his desk, etc. They are taught to do these things just so the SAS officer can maintain some level of control and psychological stability, even in an extremely bad situation.

#6: Know the Four Psychological Stages You'll Go Through When Attacked—and Try to Move through Them as Fast as You Can: When people are attacked—especially if it's fast and physical—they go through certain psychological stages as their minds try to process the events that are occurring. In fact, it's a pretty predictable process that every human goes through.

The key is not to try to change human psychology and disrupt this process. The key is to know about these stages and what's going to happen to you and then try to move through them as quickly as possible.

Why move through them as quickly as possible?

Because the end stages are where you'll have the brain power and adrenaline working for you to figure out how to escape and fight back. In the beginning stages you may be frozen and incapable of taking action.

Here are the four psychological stages most people go through when attacked:

#1: Disorientation – "What's happening to me?"

#2: Disbelief/Denial – "Is this really happening to me? / I can't BELIEVE this is happening to me!"

#3: Depression/Questioning – "Why is this happening to me? / Am I going to die? / I'm so sad this is happening to me!"

#4: Displeasure/Anger – "I'm pissed this is happening to me. / Damned if I'm going to let this happen to me!"

This last stage—the displeasure/anger stage—is the one you really want to get to as fast as possible. Not everyone gets to it. Some people end up stuck in the third stage.

But if you can, you want to do whatever it takes to get to stage #4 and take the subsequent actions you'll need to protect yourself.

I should also mention that you start to think and plan in stage #4 and beyond. You are in action mode, assessing the situation, looking for what you can do, looking for weaknesses in your attacker, etc.

Stage #4 is also where your survival instincts will kick in—in an effort to save your life.

You may have witnessed this before when hearing other people's stories of how they survived dangerous situations. In most cases, they will tell about a moment of clarity when they just knew what they had to do in order to survive.

That's the last stage, and your survival instincts are now running in full gear, helping you think clearly and remain calm. Even though you will be calm, you'll still have energy to do what you need to do. You will be alert and on top of your game. You will have the incredible power of your survival instincts, which many times are picking up on subconscious and conscious clues, putting them all together and telling you what to do.

In his excellent book *The Gift of Fear,* Gavin DeBecker tells a story of one of his clients that demonstrates this perfectly. She had been attacked and assaulted by a man who'd stalked her for days. She was lying in the bedroom after the assault. The man got up and told her not to move. He was going to the kitchen. When he came back, he said he would let her go.

Her survival instincts, however, kicked in, and she knew—she wasn't sure how—that she had to get up and walk out of her apartment. She just knew with absolute certainty that if she stayed there as he'd told her to, he would kill her.

So as he left the room, she got up and followed him quietly and then slipped out of the apartment when he was in the kitchen.

She didn't realize until later just how she knew this man was, in fact, going to kill her if she stayed in her room. Later on, she remembered this one simple fact: The man had closed her bedroom window (which had been open) moments before he told her not to move.

Her subconscious had picked up on that one simple action and told her that he was closing the bedroom window so that nobody would hear her scream. He fully intended to kill her. In fact, he had gone to the kitchen to find a knife to stab her.

By listening to her survival instincts and taking action, she'd saved her own life.

#7: Don't Blame Yourself: Throughout this book I've said that by using the ABCs of psychological self-defense, you can avoid up to 95 percent of all attacks. However, what about the other 5 percent?

What happens when you've done everything you could and you still get attacked? Don't blame yourself.

Realize that sometimes things happen that are completely beyond your control and it's not your fault. Sometimes there really isn't anything you could have done to prevent being attacked. Blaming yourself won't solve anything. The important thing is to accept the situation as it is now and start taking steps to save your life. (Remember, you still have some control.)

Try to move through the shock, disbelief, and depression you feel about finding yourself in the situation, and get to the anger and survival instincts that can help save your life. Trust that they are there—everyone has them and you're no different. They will be there for you when you need them.

This last point was demonstrated by a brave young woman who approached me after one of my seminars on personal self-protection.

She, unfortunately, had found herself in that rare 5 percent-type of situation she could not have done anything about. She'd found herself going into her apartment one night when a man appeared out of nowhere and held a knife to her throat. Her door was already open. She had no choice but to let him in, and he assaulted her.

She let him do what he wanted and then he'd left.

"What could I have done in that situation?" she asked me. "What did I do wrong?"

"Absolutely nothing," I said. "You did nothing wrong. In fact, you did everything right."

"What do you mean?" she asked.

"You're alive," I said. "You listened to your survival instincts and did what you had to do to survive—as painful as that was. You shouldn't be blaming yourself—you should be proud. You're a hero, and you survived."

Her instincts told her that in that situation she shouldn't fight back. Her instincts told her that she'd get through it and that he'd most likely leave if she let him do what he wanted. Her instincts were right—and she'd survived.

It was obviously not the outcome anyone would choose, but she survived a very bad situation where the option was to either be raped, or be raped and then killed. Sometimes life doesn't hand you very good options. She had made the best decision she could with the information she had.

Sometimes there is nothing else you could have done. Don't blame yourself. Instead, listen to your instincts, take in as much information as you can, and do what you need to do in order to survive.

Realize that you will come out of this. You are stronger than you know.

Important Points:

If a confrontation turns physical, there are still ways you can fight back and survive:

- ◊ Never let yourself be taken to a secondary location.
- ◊ If you commit to fighting back, commit to going all the way, and don't stop until the attacker cannot come after you.
- ◊ Use a distraction to give yourself time to get away.
- ◊ Make a plan ahead of time regarding what you'll do in the event of an attack and rehearse it in your mind on a regular basis.
- ◊ Realize you always have some form of control in every situation; it will keep you moving forward.
- ◊ Try to move through the four psychological emotional states that happen to everyone when attacked. Get to the last stage as soon as you can—the anger stage where you can plan, take action, and fight back.
- ◊ Don't blame yourself. Sometimes there isn't anything you could have done to prevent an attack. Accept it and ask yourself what you can do now to get out of it alive.
- ◊ Do whatever it takes to survive—you are stronger than you know.

Chapter 15 –
Finding Your Inner Warrior

By Chuck O'Neill

"Study strategy over the years and achieve the spirit of the warrior. Today is victory over yourself of yesterday; tomorrow is your victory over lesser men." — Miyamoto Musashi

"We gain strength, and courage, and confidence by each experience in which we really stop to look fear in the face...we must do that which we think we cannot." — Eleanor Roosevelt

A few years back, Kate and I had a dog named Hunter. Hunter was 120 pounds of purebred American Rottweiler. He was huge, sleek, powerful, and all muscle. He was one of the most magnificent-looking guard dogs I'd ever seen.

The problem was that Hunter didn't know he was a Rottweiler.

In his mind, he was a five-pound lap dog. All he wanted to do was cuddle. He didn't have a vicious bone in his body. He never growled, never bullied, and would happily hand over his beloved stuffed toys to anyone who asked. If you gave him an empty peanut butter jar to lick, he'd probably go home with you.

But then there was Gus.

Gus was a nine-pound Shih Tzu who ruled the dog park in our town. One nasty bark from Gus would send Hunter running for cover between my legs. My gigantic Rottweiler—who could have eaten Gus for lunch—was terrified by this fearless, confident, nine-pound 'alpha' dog. Frankly, it was embarrassing.

The thing is, I think most of us are like Hunter. We don't know the power that we have. We don't know what we're really capable of, and because of this, we find ourselves getting pushed around by bullies like Gus that we could easily walk away from.

We may feel powerless because the world has told us we're just victims: victims of predators, victims of con artists, victims of swindlers, victims of cheaters and other predators who want to use us. We live in a fear-based world, and fear can make you feel like you're powerless to protect yourself.

But the truth is that we're warriors; we just need to discover this and act on it. Hunter eventually did. There was one day—and one incident—that caused him to find his inner warrior, when it really counted.

Finding Hunter's Inner Warrior

The man was large, burly, and came to the back entrance of our house.

We had just moved into the home the week before. We didn't know that this knife-wielding criminal had tried to break in a few weeks earlier. We didn't know the previous homeowner had been forced to call the police when this man had tried to break down the door and attack her.

We didn't know that this man had been a former resident of the halfway home two streets over from us. We didn't know that he'd gotten away the first time. We didn't know that he'd decided to come back and finish the job that morning. But we'd soon find out.

I was at work. My wife was pouring her coffee in the kitchen. That was when she heard the heavy steps pounding up the back stairway. Kate had only a brief moment to wonder why an obviously large man was coming to the back door instead of the front.

That's the moment Hunter found his inner warrior.

In an instant, he went from snoring lazily under the kitchen table to fully alert and running like a demon for the back door. Hair bristling on the back of his neck, a hostile warning bark exploding from deep in his chest, Hunter drew up on his hind legs and hurled his gigantic front paws up against the back door.

Kate dropped her coffee.

She'd never seen Hunter like that. He'd never made that sound before—or even shown his teeth. He was now so large and looming that he seemed to have gained 50 pounds in less than a minute.

And he was focused with laser-like intensity on whoever was now at our back door.

Kate was far enough away that she couldn't see through the gauzy curtain over the back door window. But Hunter could. He was face-to-face with whoever was standing there. And judging by the menacing growls now rolling off his chest, he didn't like them.

Kate tried to assess the situation. Hunter had never acted this way. Strangers came to the door all the time. We'd had countless people to our home, and all Hunter had ever done was drool over them with kisses. He never even barked at the mailman.

Something was very, very wrong. Unsure what to do, Kate waited. And waited. Hunter stopped growling after a couple of minutes but still stood resolutely on his hind legs, unwilling to leave the door.

Eventually, he dropped to the floor and backed up for a better view, occasionally emitting a low growl or two. Kate then tiptoed to the back door and looked out.

The man was gone.

It was only later that we found out the whole story from the neighbours and realized the man had probably returned (not realizing the previous owner had moved) to finish the job.

We didn't know—but Hunter had known. And he'd found his inner warrior when it most counted.

I hope it doesn't take a similar situation to help you find your inner warrior. I hope this book has helped you to do the same as Hunter—to discover how strong you really are.

I hope this book has helped you find your inner warrior and prepared you to defend yourself against predators that come your way—before they attack.

By using the ABCs of Psychological Self-Defense:

◊ Awareness

◊ Body Language and Boundaries

◊ Confrontation—Verbal and Visual Skills

I believe you can stop 95 percent of attacks before they happen. You don't have to be a statistic. You can be an overcomer. You can be a warrior.

Even if you've experienced an attack in the past, I have news for you—you're already a warrior. Just the fact that you're alive, that you're here and reading this book, makes you a survivor.

Refuse to let the past rule your life. Go out and develop the skills of awareness, body language, and boundaries. Walk in the power that you have as one of God's creatures, with the right to defend yourself and win over the predators who are sizing you up every day.

Do this and I believe that just like Hunter, you will find your inner warrior. And you'll be a walking nightmare for any predator that comes your way!

Author's Note:

Thank you for reading *Psychological Self Defense*! If you found it useful, we would appreciate it so much if you would consider leaving a review of the book on Amazon. It will help others and it will be a great encouragement to us as well! Thank you!

Chuck and Kate

About the Authors

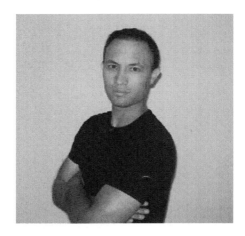

    Chuck O'Neill is a personal protection specialist, black belt martial artist, and former certified bodyguard. He is the owner of Revolution Wing Chun in Toronto, Ontario, Canada and regularly speaks to groups on personal protection and psychological self-defense.

    To learn more about Chuck, visit his websites at:

    www.SifuChuck.com

    www.LearnWingChunOnline.com

    www.RevolutionWingChun.com

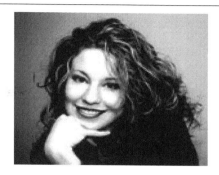

Kate O'Neill has a Bachelor of Science degree from the University of Toronto in Psychology and Human Behavior. She is a body language educator and runs the popular blog, BodyLanguageMatters.com.

To learn more visit:

www.BodyLanguageMatters.com

Appendix A: Recommended Reading

The Gift of Fear and Other Survival Signals That Protect Us from Violence. Gavin De Becker.

The Little Black Book of Violence—What Every Young Man Needs to Know about Fighting. Lawrence A. Kane and Kris Wilder.

The Sociopath Next Door. Martha Stout, PhD.

In Sheep's Clothing—Understanding and Dealing with Manipulative People. George K. Simon.

Self Defense against the Psychopath: Essential Reading for Everyone. Rik Atherton.

Without Conscience—The Disturbing World of the Psychopaths among Us. Robert D. Hare, PhD.

Boundaries—When to Say YES, When to Say NO to Take Control of Your Life. Henry Cloud and John Townsend.

What Every BODY is Saying—An Ex-FBI Agent's Guide to Speed-Reading People. Joe Navarro.

People of the Lie. M. Scott Peck.

The Survivors Club—The Secrets and Science that Could Save Your Life. Ben Sherwood.

The Definitive Book of Body Language. Allan and Barbara Pease.

Spy the Lie. Philip Houson, Michael Floyd, and Susan Carnicero.

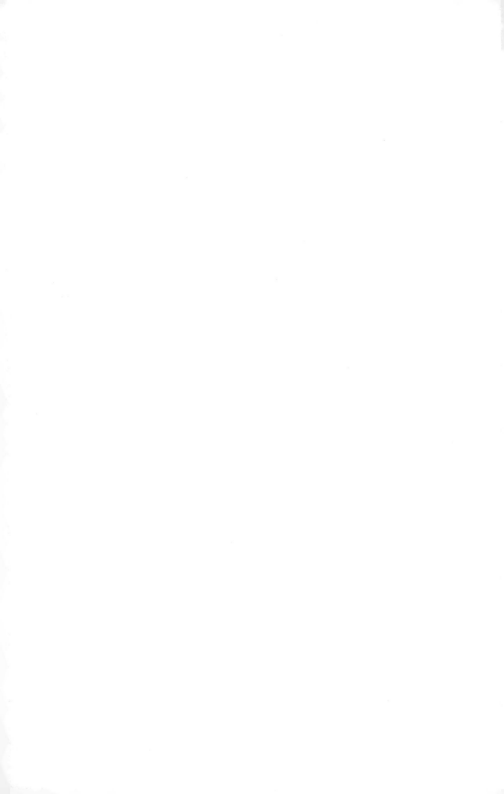

Made in the USA
Charleston, SC
04 November 2013